Degenerative Retinopathies: Advances in Clinical and Genetic Research

Proceedings of the Sixth World Congress
of the International Retinitis Pigmentosa Association (IRPA)
Dublin, Ireland
July 20 to 22, 1990

Editors

Peter Humphries, Ph.D., FTCD
Department of Genetics
Trinity College
University of Dublin
Dublin, Ireland

Shomi Bhattacharya, Ph.D.
Department of Human Genetics
University of Newcastle-upon-Tyne
Newcastle-upon-Tyne, England

Alan Bird, M.D., FRCS, FCOphth
Institute of Ophthalmology
University of London
London, England

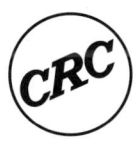

CRC Press
Boca Raton   Ann Arbor   Boston

PREFACE

This book highlights the remarkable progress in our understanding of inherited ophthalmic conditions which has been made possible by the revolution in molecular genetic techniques. At this stage, genes for a large number of X-linked heritable eye conditions have been localized, and it is worthy of note that the cloning of the gene responsible for choroideremia was reported at this symposium. Similarly, further details of the genetic mapping of the first autosomal gene responsible for the dominant form of retinitis pigmentosa (ARDP) were reported. It has been established that a proportion of ADRP families map to the long arm of chromosome 3 and that other families do not show genetic linkage to this region of the human genome, demonstrating genetic heterogeneity. Our ability to amplify target sequences by the polymerase chain reaction and to directly analyze mutations by sequencing has resulted in the extraordinary finding of a single amino acid substitution (a proline-histidine at codon 23) in the rhodopsin gene of some ADRP patients. Other rhodopsin mutations were also reported at this congress.

The involvement of rhodopsin, a key element of the visual transduction pathway, raises interesting and exciting possibilities for the involvement of the other components of the pathway (e.g., transducin or phosphodiesterase) or the photoreceptor cytoskeleton (e.g., peripherin) as candidates for the many different forms of retinal degeneration in man. Both phosphodiesterase (PDE) and peripherin have been implicated in the *rd* and *rds* mutations in mice. Furthermore, Usher syndrome (Type 1) — a recessive form of retinitis pigmentosa along with congenital deafness — has been mapped to the long arm of chromosome 1 by genetic linkage analysis.

The Sixth World Congress of the International Retinitis Pigmentosa Association (IRPA) served to condense many of these exciting developments and at a most appropriate time, as the chapters in this book admirably demonstrate. We are now well into the era of "reverse genetics" which will soon result in the identification of many, if not all, inherited retinopathy genes. We may be certain that such knowledge will contribute profoundly to the diagnosis and eventual therapy of this important group of degenerative retinal diseases.

Peter Humphries
Shomi S. Bhattacharya
Alan C. Bird

CONTRIBUTORS

M. Abitbol
Centre Hospitalier Universitaire Necker
 Enfants Malades
INSERM
Paris, France

M. Abraham
Medical Research Foundation
Madras, India

L. Alonso
Department of Ophthalmology
Clinic Hospital
Valencia, Spain

C. Lynn Anson-Cartwright
Department of Genetics
The Research Institute
The Hospital for Sick Children
Toronto, Ontario, Canada

B. N. Apte
Medical Genetic Unit
Bombay Hospital
Bombay, India

A. Avakian
Edward S. Harkness Eye Institute
Columbia University
New York, New York

A. Awad-Michel
Centre Hospitalier Universitaire Necker
 Enfants Malades
Paris, France

R. Bashir
Molecular Genetics Unit
University of Newcastle-upon-Tyne
Newcastle-upon-Tyne, England

M. Beneyto
Department of Genetics
La Fe Hospital
Valencia, Spain

S. S. Bhattacharya
Department of Human Genetics
University of Newcastle-upon-Tyne
Newcastle-upon-Tyne, England

A. C. Bird
Institute of Ophthalmology
University of London
London, England

Graeme Black
The Genetics Laboratory
Department of Biochemistry
University of Oxford
Oxford, England

Susan H. Blanton
Medical Genetics Center
University of Texas Health Science
 Center
Houston, Texas

J. Boix
Department of Ophthalmology
Clinic Hospital
Valencia, Spain

D. Bonneau
Service de Pédiatrie
Centre Hospitalier Universitaire
Poitiers, France

R. Bosch
Department of Ophthalmology
Clinic Hospital
Valencia, Spain

D. G. Bradley
Department of Genetics
Trinity College
Dublin, Ireland

M. L. Briard
INSERM U. 12
Unité de Recherches sur les Handicaps
 Génétiques de l'Enfant
Hôpital des Enfants Malades
Paris, France

Arthur H. M. Burghes
Departments of Molecular Genetics,
 Physiological Chemistry, and Neurology
University of Ohio
Columbus, Ohio

A. Chand
Department of Biochemistry
University of Otago
Dunedin, New Zealand
 and Department of Pathology
Prince of Wales Hospital
Sydney, Australia

Zhengyi Chen
The Genetics Laboratory
Department of Biochemistry
University of Oxford
Oxford, England

V. Colantuoni
Dipartimento di Biochimica e
 Biotechnologie Mediche
Universita di Napoli
Napoli, Italy

Anne Cottingham
Medical Genetics Center
University of Texas Health Science
 Center
Houston, Texas

Ian Craig
The Genetics Laboratory
Department of Biochemistry
University of Oxford
Oxford, England

F. Cremers
Institute of Human Genetics
Nijmegen, The Netherlands

Sandra Pieke Dahl
Boys Town National Research Hospital
Omaha, Nebraska

Stephen P. Daiger
Medical Genetics Center
University of Texas Health Science
 Center
Houston, Texas

A. David
Service de Pédiatrie
Centre Hospitalier Universitaire
Nantes, France

M. Del Bo
Institute of Audiology
University of Milan
Milan, Italy

M. J. Denton
Department of Biochemistry
University of Otago
Dunedin, New Zealand

J. Du
Edward S. Harkness Eye Institute
Columbia University
New York, New York

J. L. Dufier
Centre Hospitalier Universitaire Necker
 Enfants Malades
INSERM
 and Consultation d'Ophtalmologie
Hôpital Laënnec
Paris, France

G. J. Farrar
Department of Genetics
Trinity College
Dublin, Ireland

Yijian Fei
Department of Ophthalmology
The First University Hospital
West China University of Medical
 Sciences
Chengdu, China

G. Fishman
Department of Ophthalmology
Eye and Ear Hospital
Chicago, Illinois

R. Forte
University of Rome "La Sapienza"
Institute of Ophthalmology
Rome, Italy

J. Frezal
Centre Hospitalier Universitaire Necker
 Enfants Malades
  and INSERM U. 12 Unité de
  Recherches sur les Handicaps
  Génétiques de l'Enfant
Hôpital des Enfants Malades
Paris, France

Keiko Fujiki
Department of Ophthalmology
Juntendo University School of Medicine
Tokyo, Japan

L. Fusi
Labortorio Analisi
Ospdale Mauriziano
Torino, Italy

D. K. Gahlot
Taparia Institute of Ophthalmology
Bombay Hospital
Bombay, India

A. Gal
Institüt für Humangenetik der Universität
Bonn and Lübeck, Germany

F. B. Gibberd
Consultant Neurologist
Westminster Hospital
London, England

S. Gilgenkrantz
CRTS
Nancy, France

P. Gouras
Edward S. Harkness Eye Institute
Columbia University
New York, New York

P. Grimaldos
Department of Ophthalmology
Clinic Hospital
Valencia, Spain

V. Gualandri
Institute of Human Genetics
University of Milan
Milan, Italy

G. Guasconi
INSERM U. 12
Unité de Recherches sur les Handicaps
  Génétiques de l'Enfant
Hôpital des Enfants Malades
Paris, France

Eli Hatchwell
The Genetics Laboratory
Department of Biochemistry
University of Oxford
Oxford, England

Mutsuko Hayakawa
Department of Ophthalmology
Juntendo University School of Medicine
Tokyo, Japan

John R. Heckenlively
Jules Stein Eye Institute
University of California
Los Angeles, California

J. Fielding Hejtmancik
Baylor College of Medicine
Houston, Texas

Yoshihiro Hotta
Department of Ophthalmology
Juntendo University School of Medicine
Tokyo, Japan

Yongzhi Huang
Department of Ophthalmology
The First University Hospital
West China University of Medical
  Sciences
Chengdu, China

A. E. Hughes
Department of Medical Genetics
The Queen's University of Belfast
Belfast, Northern Ireland

M. M. Humphries
Department of Genetics
Trinity College
Dublin, Ireland

P. Humphries
Department of Genetics
Trinity College
Dublin, Ireland

A. Iannaccone
University of Rome "La Sapienza"
Institute of Ophthalmology
Rome, Italy

C. F. Inglehearn
Molecular Genetics Unit
University of Newcastle-upon-Tyne
Newcastle-upon-Tyne, England

P. Ivorra
Department of Ophthalmology
Clinic Hospital
Valencia, Spain

M. Jay
Moorfields Eye Hospital
London, England

Kazuyuki Kabasawa
Division of Information Sciences
Central Laboratory of Medical Sciences
Juntendo University School of Medicine
Tokyo, Japan

Atsushi Kanai
Department of Ophthalmology
Juntendo University School of Medicine
Tokyo, Japan

J. Kaplan
Centre Hospitalier Universitaire Necker
  Enfants Malades
    and INSERM U. 12 Unité de
    Recherches sur les Handicaps
    Génétiques de l'Enfant
Hôpital des Enfants Malades
Paris, France

Kazuo Kato
Department of Opthalmology
Juntendo University School of Medicine
Tokyo, Japan

D. Kauffmann
Edward S. Harkness Eye Institute
Columbia University
New York, New York

J. Keen
Molecular Genetics Unit
University of Newcastle-upon-Tyne
Newcastle-upon-Tyne, England

Paul F. Kenna
Department of Genetics
Trinity College
  and Research Department
Royal Victoria Eye and Ear Hospital
Dublin, Ireland

Judith B. Kenyon
Boys Town National Research Hospital
Omaha, Nebraska

William J. Kimberling
Boys Town National Research Hospital
Omaha, Nebraska

H. Kjeldbye
Edward S. Harkness Eye Institute
Columbia University
New York, New York

G. Kumaramanickavel
Institute of Physiology and Experimental
  Medicine
Madras Medical College
Madras, India

R. Kwun
Edward S. Harkness Eye Institute
Columbia University
New York, New York

Jana Laidlaw
Medical Genetics Center
University of Texas Health Science
  Center
Houston, Texas

B. Lauffart
Molecular Genetics Unit
University of Newcastle-upon-Tyne
Newcastle-upon-Tyne, England

D. Lester
Molecular Genetics Unit
University of Newcastle-upon-Tyne
Newcastle-upon-Tyne, England

Anren Li
Department of Ophthalmology
The First University Hospital
West China University of Medical
  Sciences
Chengdu, China

R. Lopez
Edward S. Harkness Eye Institute
Columbia University
New York, New York

Birgit Lorenz
Augenklinik
Universität München
München, Germany

Chengren Luo
Department of Ophthalmology
The First University Hospital
West China University of Medical
  Sciences
Chengdu, China

C. Marchese
Labortorio Analisi
Ospdale Mauriziano
Torino, Italy

Alessandro Martini
University of Padova
Padova, Italy

Cathy McDowell
Department of Genetics
The Research Institute
The Hospital for Sick Children
Toronto, Ontario, Canada

P. McWilliam
Department of Genetics
Trinity College
Dublin, Ireland

Thomas Meitinger
Abteilung für Paediatrische Genetik
Kinderpoliklinik der Universität München
München, Germany

J. Melki
INSERM U. 12
Unité de Recherches sur les Handicaps
  Genetique de l'Enfant
Hôpital des Enfants Malades
Paris, France

Massimo Milani
University of Padova
Padova, Italy

Claes Moller
University of Linköping
Linköping, Sweden

A. Munnich
INSERM U. 12
Unité de Recherches sur les Handicaps
  Génétiques de l'Enfant
Hôpital des Enfants Malades
Paris, France

Maria A. Musarella
Department of Genetics
The Research Institute and Department of
  Ophthalmology
The Hospital for Sick Children
Toronto, Ontario, Canada

Akira Nakajima
Department of Opthalmology
Juntendo University School of Medicine
Tokyo, Japan

Atsuo Nakamura
Department of Ophthalmology
Juntendo University School of Medicine
Tokyo, Japan

Larry Overbeck
Boys Town National Research Hospital
Omaha, Nebraska

B. Page
Department of Ophthalmology
The Queen's University of Belfast
Belfast, Northern Ireland

L. Pannarale
University of Rome "La Sapienza"
Institute of Ophthalmology
Rome, Italy

M. R. Pannarale
University of Rome "La Sapienza"
Institute of Ophthalmology
Rome, Italy

S. S. Papiha
Molecular Genetics Unit
University of Newcastle-upon-Tyne
Newcastle-upon-Tyne, England

I. H. Pawlowiski
Institute for Human Genetics
Münster, Germany

Mary Z. Pelias
Louisiana State University Medical
  Center
New Orleans, Louisiana

F. Piattoni
Institute of Human Genetics
University of Milan
Milan, Italy

C. Pierrottet
Department of Ophthalmology
University of Milan
Milan, Italy

J. Pongratz
Institüt für Humangenetik der Universität
Bonn and Lübeck, Germany

A. Porta
Department of Ophthalmology
University of Milan
Milan, Italy

John Powell
The Genetics Laboratory
Department of Biochemistry
University of Oxford
Oxford, England

F. Prieto
Department of Genetics
La Fe Hospital
Valencia, Spain

R. Redmond
Departments of Ophthalmology and
  Medical Genetics
The Queen's University of Belfast
  and City Hospital
Belfast, Northern Ireland

Susan Riley
The Genetics Laboratory
Department of Biochemistry
University of Oxford
Oxford, England

E. Rispoli
University of Rome "La Sapienza"
Institute of Ophthalmology
Rome, Italy

Joseph A. Rodriguez
Medical Genetics Center
University of Texas Health Science
  Center
Houston, Texas

Johanna M. Rommens
Department of Genetics
The Research Institute
The Hospital for Sick Children
Toronto, Ontario, Canada

H. H. Ropers
Institute of Human Genetics
Nijmegen, The Netherlands

Ch. Samanns
Institüt für Humangenetik der Universität
Bonn and Lübeck, Germany

P. Sforza
Edward S. Harkness Eye Institute
Columbia University
New York, New York

E. M. Sharp
Department of Genetics
Trinity College
Dublin, Ireland

Yin Y. Shugart
Boys Town National Research Hospital
Omaha, Nebraska

Ole Sjö
Division of Paediatric Ophthalmology and
  Handicaps
Gentofte Hospital
Gentofte, Denmark

Richard J. H. Smith
Baylor College of Medicine
Houston, Texas

G. Staurenghi
Department of Ophthalmology
University of Milan
Milan, Italy

Utako Tanabe
Department of Ophthalmology
Juntendo University School of Medicine
Tokyo, Japan

Lisbeth Tranebjærg
Department of Medical Genetics
The John F. Kennedy Institute
Glostrup, Denmark

L. Troiano
Institute of Audiology
University of Milan
Milan, Italy

C. Vilela
Department of Neurophysiology
La Fe Hospital
Valencia, Spain

E. M. Vingolo
University of Rome "La Sapienza"
Insitute of Ophthalmology
Rome, Italy

Mette Warburg
Division of Paediatric Ophthalmology and
  Handicaps
Gentofte Hospital
Gentofte, Denmark

A. Watty
Institüt für Humangenetik der Universität
Bonn, Germany

Michael D. Weston
Boys Town National Research Hospital
Omaha, Nebraska

Robert Williamson
Department of Molecular Genetics
St. Mary's Hospital Medical School
University of London
London, England

Baerbel Wittwer
Institüt für Medizinische Genetik am
  Bezirkskrankenhaus Magdeburg
Magdeburg, Germany

Jiumu Zhou
Department of Ophthalmology
The First University Hospital
West China University of Medical
  Sciences
Chengdu, China

TABLE OF CONTENTS

STUDY OF FAMILIES WITH RETINITIS PIGMENTOSA
IN THE GEOGRAPHIC AREA OF VALENCIA (SPAIN)

L.Alonso*, P.Grimaldos*, J.Boix*, R.Bosch*,
P.Ivorra*, C.Vilela**, F.Prieto***, M.Beneyto***

* CLINIC HOSPITAL (VALENCIA)-OPHTHALMOLOGY
** LA FE HOSPITAL (VALENCIA)-NEUROPHYSIOLOGY
*** LA FE HOSPITAL (VALENCIA)-GENETICS

I. SUMMARY

In this study we have investigated a total of 92 patients with R.P. from 61 families. Ophthalmological explorations have been carried out on all of them, including computerized perimetry and electrophysiological tests. Pedigree structures for each family, over three to four generations, have been compiled.

Out of the 61 families studied we find 13.1% present as autosomal dominant, 34.4% we find recessive R.P. and 1.6% as X-linked. We were unable to establish the type of inheritance in 50.8% of cases, classifying these as sporadic or simplex.

We have also studied the average age of appearance of symptoms in each genetic type, the incidence of cataracts and the seriousness of the illness.

II. INTRODUCTION

R.P. is defined as a combination of progressive degeneration of the retina which affects the rod and cone cells and the pigment epithelium layer. It has a frequency of between 1/300 and 1/5000 , being the fourth most prevalent cause of blindness in the world. Approximate 50% of cases are hereditary, transmission being either autosomal dominant, recessive or X-linked.

In this comparative study we have investigated the incidence in Valencia (Spain) of each genetic type, and the relationship between the disease and the appearance of cataracts.

III. METHODS

Ninety two patients with R.P., belonging to sixty one families were investigated. Details, including initial symptoms, actual symptoms, age at which symptoms had appeared, progression and relapse of the disease, visual acuity, optical correction, fundus examination and biomicroscopy were noted. A Farnsworth colour test was performed on all patients. Computerized perimetry (after 20 minutes of dark adaptation) using the Octopus 500 and using the short test program is shown in Figure 1. Other explorations carried out were: direct and indirect ophthalmoscopy, simple retinography, electrophysiological tests (consisting in the performance of ERG after 45 minutes of adaptation to darkness using blue and white light (Figure 2)) and visual and auditive evoked potentials.

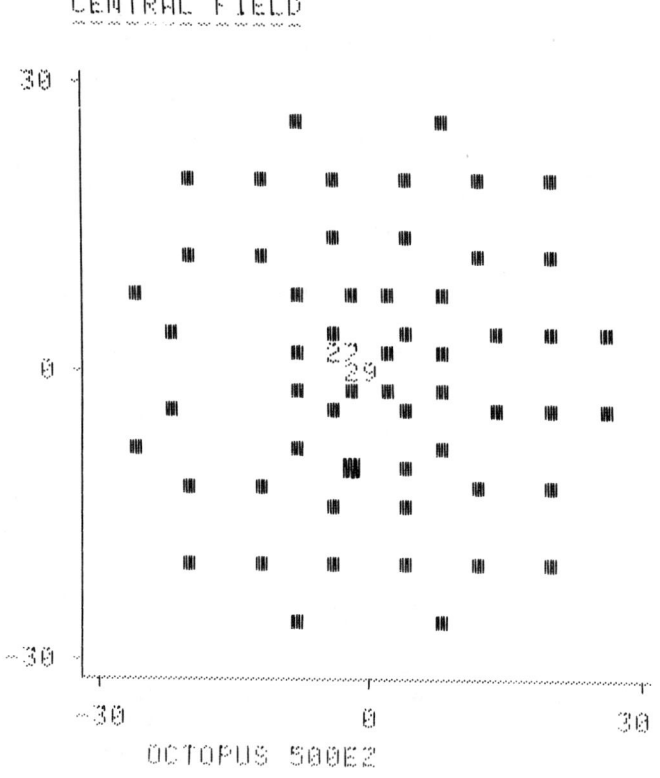

Figure 1. Affected patient computerized perimetry

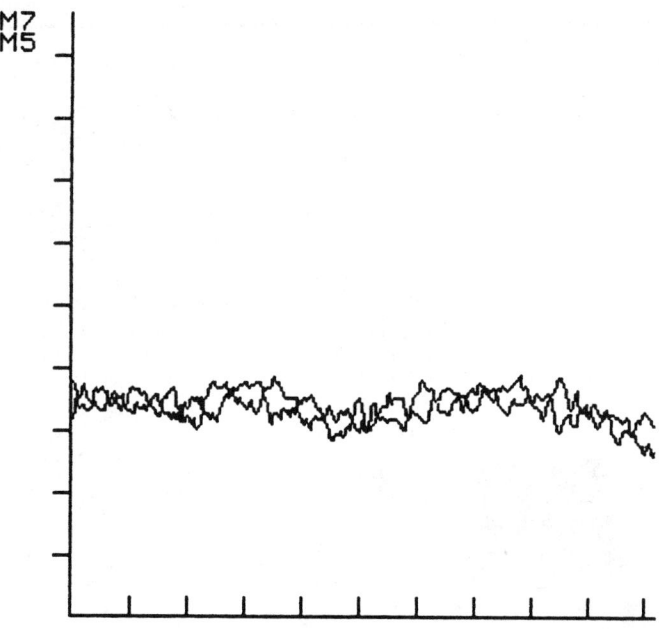

Figure 2. Affected patient ERG

The disease was genetically assessed as autosomal dominant when the pedigree showed a linear transmission of the illness (parents to children) and a segregation ratio of around 0.4%.

The disease was classed as autosomal recessive when linear transmission did not exist. Lastly the disease was classified as sporadic or simplex, when no relative was affected.

IV. RESULTS

The first result obtained was the genetic distribution of R.P., finding in the 61 families the following percentage (Figure 3): 1-Autosomal Recessive: 34.4%; 2-Autosomal Dominant: 13.1%; 3- X-linked: 1.6% 4- Sporadic or Simplex: 50.8%.

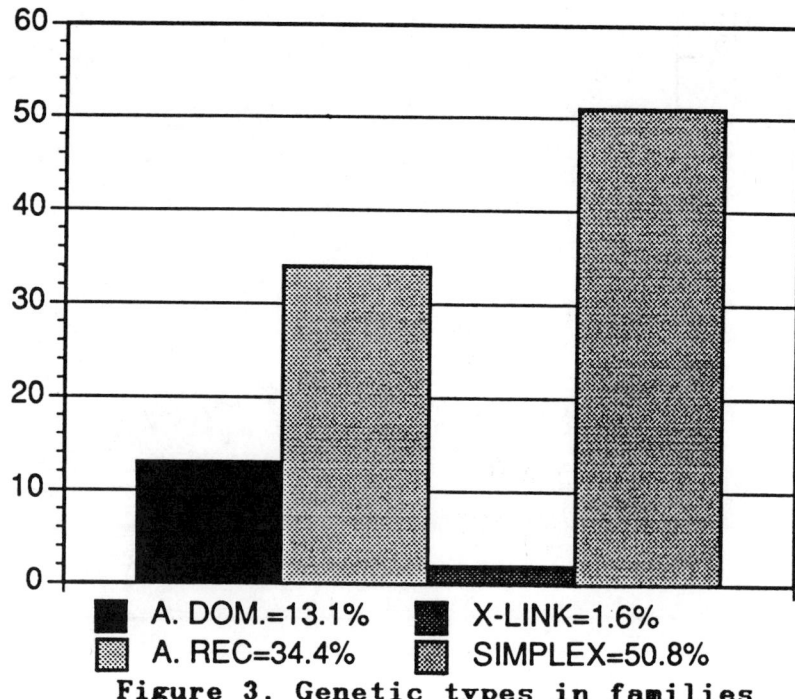

Figure 3. Genetic types in families

The frequency of genetic distribution obtained in the study of 92 patients shown in Figure 4. is as follows: 1- autosomal recessive: 35.8%; 2- autosomal dominant: 26%; 3- X-linked: 4.3% 4- sporadic or simplex: 33.6%.

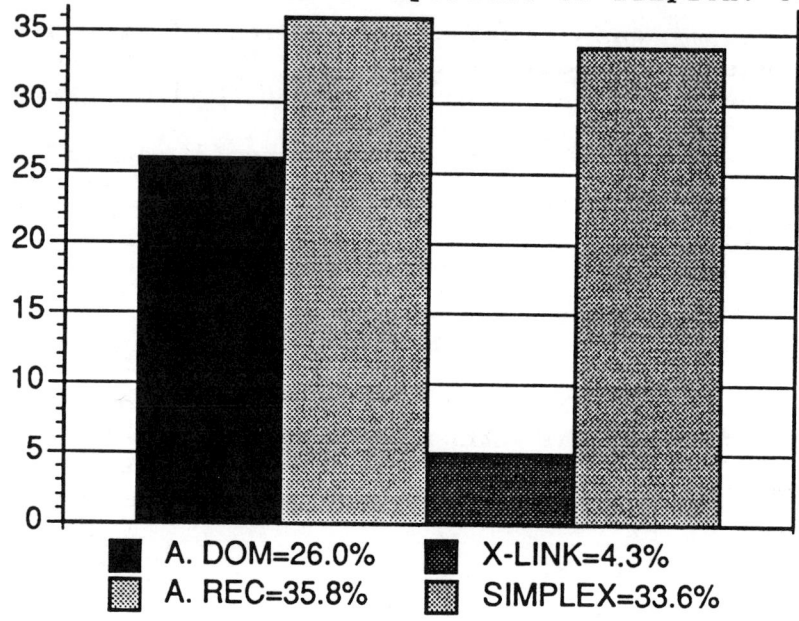

Figure 4. - Genetic types in patients

Once the genetic distribution was obtained,we related

this with :

A. Age of appearance of symptoms:

Symptoms, such as night blindness, bumping into objects
and subjective loss of visual field, appear in more than
60% of patients before reaching the age of 20 in
autosomal dominant, recessive and sporadic cases. In the
rest before the age of 40. Nevertheless in X-linked
inheritance, symptoms appear in 100% of patients before
reaching the age of 10 .

B. Appearance of cataracts:

We have observed an important relationship between the
appearance of cataracts and R.P., finding that it
appeared in 46% of patients in the autosomal dominant
form, in 54% of autosomal recessive, in 80% of sporadic
and in 100% of X-linked cases (Figure 5). We also
observe that 100% of patients over 50 years of age
develop cataracts, regardless of the genetic type, these
being of posterior subcapsular type.

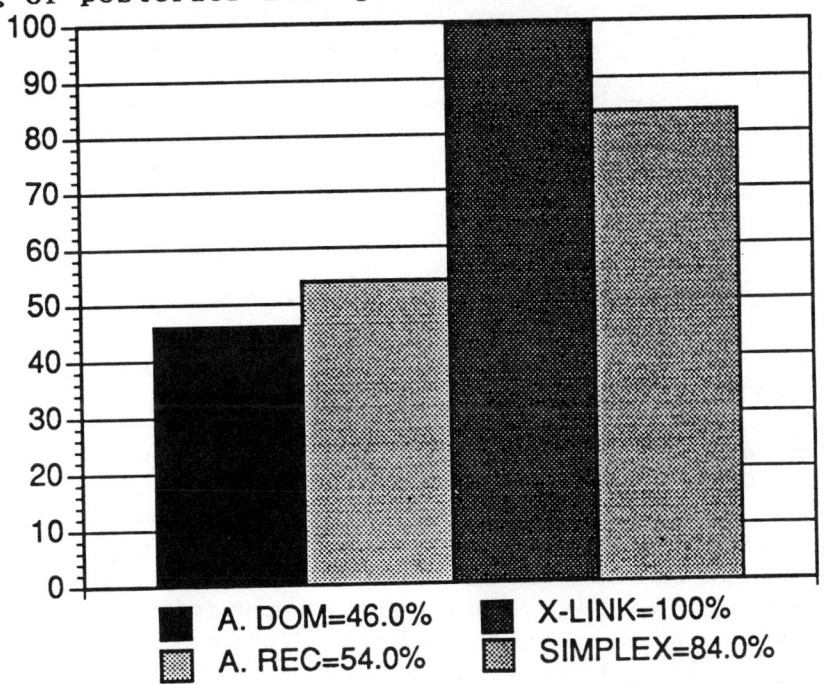

Figure 5. Incidence of cataract in R.P. genetic types

C. Seriousness of illness:

We find that of the total number of patients, 19% are proclaimed unfit to carry out their previous jobs due to R.P. Regarding the relation with genetic distribution we observe 50% of X-linked patients were declared unfit for their previous professions, in sporadic cases 26%, in autosomal recessive 24%, and lastly 10% in the cases of autosomal dominant inheritance. Finally we observed that when the illness is further advanced, patients show a more serious situation in that 78% with severe clinical symptoms have been affected for over 15 years.

V. DISCUSSION

Observing our results on the genetic distribution in other families affected with R.P. and comparing them with other authors (Table 1) the results can be seen to coincide in sporadic cases which show maximum incidence. The X-linked form shows the minimum incidence except as reported by Bird.

	PAGON (1)	BOUGHMAN (3)	BIRD (4)	FISHMAN (5)	HEREDIA (6)	VALENCIA
Autosomal Dominant	15-25	20	26	19	6	13
Autosomal Recessive	5-20	16	13	19	27	34
X-linked	5-15	12	22	8	4	2
Simplex	40-50	41	43	52	63	51

Table 1. Genetic types of families. Comparison with other authors.

In the autosomal recessive form we find the same as Heredia (6), i.e., a higher incidence than in the autosomal dominant form, contrary to other studies carried out by Anglosaxon authors. Hence, other genetic factors might exist which in some way influence the distribution. We have also related genetic distribution in patients with other authors (Table 2) noting the similarity with frequencies shown in the study by Heredia (6). In the study by Dickinson (7) (Table 2) the absence of sporadic cases shows up, this is due to the fact that he attributes an autosomal recessive inheritance to sporadic cases, as do other authors, such as Seiff (8). In the geographic area were we have carried out our investigation a predominance of the hereditary pattern of autosomal recessive is observed both in the study of patients and of families.

	FISHMAN (5)	BOUGHMAN (3)	DICKINSON (7)	HEREDIA (6)	VALENCIA
Autosomal Dominant	26	22	27	12	26
Autosomal Recessive	19	16	62	37	36
X-linked	16	9	11	6	4
Simplex	38	50	--	45	34

Table 2.- Genetic types in Spain, in comparison with other authors.

Regarding the age at which symptoms appear, we note that X-linked cases are the earliest, appearing before 10 years of age, observations coinciding with authors such as Heredia (6) and Wolf (9). Although contrary to these authors we do not find any difference regarding the age at which symptoms appear between autosomal dominant and recessive forms.

The relation between R.P. and the appearance of cataracts is evident and this is noted in 100% of patients over 50 years of age. Observations in which 100% of patients with X-linked R.P. show cataracts, coincide with studies by Fishman (5).

This last conclusion could follow variations in other studies as the sample for these inherited X-linked cases, in our study is very reduced. We also believe as Fishman (5), that the cataract is not the most important cause for the decresase of visual acuity but is due to alterations in the retina.

Regarding a correlation between severity and genetic type, our observations coincide with the majority of authors, in that the most serious form is X-linked, followed by autosomal recessive and finally the less severe, autosomal dominant form. Regarding sporadic or simplex forms, these show a similar seriousness to autosomal recessive, which would warrant the inclusion of these patients in the recessive form by authors such as Dickinson (7) and Seiff (8). Therefore we describe in our investigation the great importance of R.P. both for the patients who suffer and for their families and social circles, due to the unfortunate prognosis of the illness and the present lack of efficient treatment.

VI. CONCLUSIONS

A.- R.P. appears in our geographic area with the following genetic distribution:

1.- Autosomal dominant: 34.4%
2.- Autosomal recessive: 13.1%
3.- X-linked: 1.6%
4.- Sporadic or simplex: 50.8%

B.- R.P. is associated with cataracts in 100% of the cases in patients over 50 years of age, regardless of genetic type.

C.- The most serious genetic form of R.P. is the X-linked and the least serious is the autosomal dominant.

VII. REFERENCES

1. Pagon,R.A. Retinitis Pigmentosa, Surv. Ophthalm., 33/3, 77-137, 1988
2. Jay, B. Hereditary aspects of R.P. Trans. Ophthalm. Soc. U.K., 92, 173-178,1978
3. Boughman, A.C., Fishman,S.A. A genetic analysis of R.P. Brit. J. Ophthalm., 67/7, 449-454, 1983
4. Bird,A.C. X-linked R.P., Brit. J. Ophthalm., 59, 177-179, 1975
5. Fishman,G.A., Retinitis Pigmentosa, Arch. Ophthalm. Chicago., 96, 822-826, 1978
6. Heredia,C.D., Engel,P., Cols,.N and Garcia Calderon,P.A. Distribución genética en pacientes con Retinosis Pigmentaria, Arch. So. Esp. Oftal., 50, 129-134, 1986
7. Dickinson,P., Mulhall,L., A survey of hereditary aspects of Pigmentary Retinal Distrophies, Aust N-Z. J. Ophthalm., 17(3), 247-256, 1989
8. Seiff,S.R., Heckenlivery,R., and Pearlman,J.T., Assesing the risk 2 of Retinitis Pigmentosa with age of onset of data, Amer. J. Ophthalm., 94, 30-43, 1982
9. Wolf,M.C., Bergsman,D.R, and Krill,A.E, Retinitis Pigmentosa Brit. Defects Compedium, New York, McMillan Press, 936-937. 1979

CHOROIDEREMIA AND OVARIAN DYSGENESIS ASSOCIATED WITH AN X ; 7 DE NOVO BALANCED TRANSLOCATION

M. ABITBOL[1], J. KAPLAN[1], S. GILGENKRANTZ[2], A. AWAD-MICHEL[1],
H.H. ROPERS[3], F. CREMERS[3], I.H. PAWLOWISKI[4], J. FREZAL[1], J.L. DUFIER[1]

(1) CHU NECKER ENFANTS MALADES - PARIS (France)
(2) CRTS NANCY (France)
(3) Institut of Human Genetics, NIJMEGEN (The Netherlands)
(4) Institut for Human Genetics MUNSTER (Germany)

I. INTRODUCTION

There are now a number of reports of de novo balanced X/autosome translocations associated with the sporadic expression of X-linked disorders in females.

- At least 20 cases of clinical Duchenne or Becker muscular dystrophy with a breakpoint at Xp21, enabling the localisation of the DMD locus at Xp21. From one of them, the X;A junction fragment was cloned and coding sequences of the DMD gene were isolated (Verellen et al, Burghes et al). Recently, 12 translocation breakpoints in the Xp21 region have been mapped (Boyd et al).

- Aicardi Syndrome with t(X;3)(p22;q12), Ropers et al.
- Aarskog Syndrome with t(X;8)(q13;21.2), Bawle et al.
- Ectodermal dysplasia with t(X;9)(q13;p21). A cell line was avalaible in the Camden catalog but it was unknown that it came from this case. Several multipoint analyses were made in order to locate the ED gene on chromosome X. They lead to the same breakpoint, Xq21.1., Zonana et al.
- Lowe Syndrome with t(X;3)(q25;27), Hodgson et al.
- Hunter Syndrome with t(X;5), Mossman et al.

As to the several cases of Incontinentia Pigmenti (IP) with translocations (X;A) involving breakpoints at Xp11, linkage analysis in extended families with IP showed that the IP gene could not be mapped at Xp11 but was actually at Xq. The associations between IP and various breakpoints upon the X chromosome is not yet fully explained, Sefiani et al.

We report the first case of chroideremia in a girl with a t(X;7(q21;p14). The break at Xq21 corresponds to the site of the choroideremia gene but is also responsible to gonadal dysgenesis.

II. CASE REPORT

A girl born in 1965 was found to have a choroideremia and a primary amenorrhea.

She was the third child and had been born at term. At birth, her father and mother were both 25 years old. Growth and development were normal. When she was 8 years old, a nyctalopia appeared associated with myopia. At 14, no sexual development appeared and **ovarian dysgenesis with streak gonads** was observed at coelioscopy. Her two sisters had a normal sexual development.

When we saw this patient she was a 24 year old woman ; she had a height of 175 cm and a weight of 70 kgs. She did not have any Turner'sign. Her **ocular findings were consistent with the diagnosis of choroideremia** : both fundis showed characteristic peripheral loss of choriocapillaris and retinal pigment epithelium except in the foveal region and sparing of the inner retina. The mother's ocular fundis was normal.

Her visual fields were lightly constricted and there was a big reduction in amplitude of both scotopic ans photopic electroretinographic responses.

Her visual acuity with correction of myopia was :

RE : 20/25

LE : 20/25

Cytogenetic studies showed from lymphocyte culture in GTG, QFQ, RBA bandings a **reciprocal translocation between Xq and 7p.** The chromosome constitution was 46,X,t (X;7) (Xpter - Xq21.2 :: 7p14 - 7pter ; Xqter -Xq21.2 :: 7p14 - 7pter). Normal X was inactived non-randomly. Parents and oldest sister had a normal karyotype.

III. DISCUSSION

Choroideremia (MCK 30310) is an X-linked retinal dystrophy and causes central blindness in affected males.

Several linkage analyses in families with this disease showed the locus was located to Xq13q21 with RLP : DXYS1 (Nussbaum et al 1985), DXS3 and DXS11 (Gall et al 1986) DXS1 and DXS17 (Lesko et al 1987)

In a Danish family, a study with pDP34 and S21 (locus DXS1) revealed and interstitial deletion associated with a tapetoretinal dystrophy in a retarded boy (Schwartz et al 1986). In a English family with a rearrangement including a deletion of sub-band Xq21.1 and a choroideremia in a male, DXYS1 and DXS3 were absent (Hodgson et al).

Recently from two other families with and interstitial deletion and choroideremia, Nussbaum et al succeded to generate a library of cloned DNA from the Xq21 segment containing the choroideremia locus by means of the phenol-enhanced reassociation technique.

Some affected boys have been shown to carry an interstitial deletion in the Xq21 region and we think the study of our breakpoint could help for identifying the segment containing the choroideremia gene and for producing junctional DNA intragenic segments.

VI. REFERENCES

1 - AYAZIZ, Choroideremia, obesity and congenital deafness, Am J Ophtalmo 92, 6369, 1981.

2 - BAWLE E, TYRKUS M, LIPMAN S, BOZIMOWSKI D, Aarskog Syndrome : full male and female expression associated with an X autosome translocation. Am J Med Genet. 17, 595-602.,1984.

3 - BOYD Y, COCKBURN D, HOLT S, MUNRO E, VAN OMMEN GJ, GILLARD B, ALLARA N, FERGUSON-SMITH M, CRAIG I, Mapping of 12 translocation breakpoints in the Xp21 region with respect ot the locus of Duchenne muscular dystrophy. Cytogenet Cell Genet, 48, 28-34.,1988.

4 - BURGHES AHM, LOGAN G, HUX X, BELFALL B, WORTON RG, RAY PN, A cDNA clone from the muscular dystrophy gene.Nature, 328, 434-437.,1987.

5 - CREMERS FPM, BRUNSMANN F, VAN DE POL TJR, PAWLOWITZKI IH, PAULSEN K, WIERINGA B, ROPERS, Deletion of the DXS165 Locus in patients with classical choroideremia.Clin Genet 92, 421-423.,1987.

6 - CREMERS FPM, VAN DE POL TJR, WIERINGA B, BRUNSMANN F, NUSSBAUM RL, ROPERS HH, Physical fine mapping of the choroideremia gene region at Xp21 in patients with syndromic or classical tapetochoroidal dystrophy (TCD). Clin Genet 34, 312.,1988.

7 - CREMERS FPM VAN DE POL TJR, WIERINGA B, BRUNSMANN F, NUSSBAUM RL, ROPERS HH, Molecular characterization of submicroscopic Xq21 deletions in patients with syndromic or classical tapetochoroidal dystrophy (TCD). Amer J Hum Genet, 43 (abstr n°718).,1988.

8 - GAL A, BRUNSMANN F, HOGENKAMP D, RUTHER K, AHLERT D, Choroideremia, -locus maps between DXS3 and DXS11 on Xq. Hum Genet, 73, 123-126.,1986.

9 - HODGSON SV, HECKMATT JZ, HUGHES E, CROLLA JA, DUBOWITZ V, BOBROW M, A balanced de novo X/autosome translocation in a girl with manifestation of Lowe Syndrome. Am J Med Genet, 23, 837-847.,1986a.

10 - HODGSON SV, ROBERTSON ME, FEAR CN, GOODSHIP J, MALCOLM S, JAY B, BOBROW M, PEMBREY ME, Prenatal diagnosis of X linked choroideremia with mental retardation associated with a cytogenetically detectable X-chromosome deletion. Hum Genet, 75, 286-290.,1987.

11 - LESKO JG, LEWIS RA, FERRELL R, NUSSBAUM RL, Choroideremia is tightly linked to two proximal Xq chromosomal markers. Am J Hum Genet, 37, suppl : A65.,1985.

12 - LESKO JG, LEWIS RA, NUSSBAUM RL, Multipoint kinkage analysis of loci in the proximal long arm of the human X chromosome : application to mapping the choroideremia locus. Am J Hum GENET, 40, 303-311.1987.

13 - LEWIS RA, NUSSBAUM RL, FERRELL R, Mapping X-linked ophthalmic diseases : provisional assignment of the locus for choroideremia to Xq13-24. Ophthalmology, 92, 800-805.,1985.

14 - MAUTHNER L, Ein Fall von Choroideremia.Naturwissenshaft Med Verein, 2, 191.1987.

15 - Mc CULLOCH C, Mc CULLOCH RPJP, A hereditary and clinical study of choroideremia. Trans Am Acad Ophthalmol Otolaryngol, 52, 160-190.1984.

16 - MERRY DE, SOSNOSKI DM, LESKO JG, COLLINS FS, LEWIS RA, NUSSBAUM RL, Chromosome jumping from DXS232 and DXS233 toward the choroideremia locus. J Hum Genet 43 (abstr n°780).,1988.

17 -   HOSSMAN J, BLUNT S, STEPHENS R, JONES EE, PEMBREY M, Hunster's disease in a girl association with (X;5) chromosomal translocation disrupting the Unter gene. Arch Dis Child, 58, 911-915.,1983.

18 -   NUSSBAUM RL, LEWIS RAN LESKO JG, FERRELL R, Choroideremia is linked to the restriction fragment length polymorphism DXYS2 at Xq13-21. Am J Hum Genet, 37, 473-481., 1985.

19 -   NUSSBAUM RL, LESKO JG, LEWIS RA, LEDBETTER SA, LEDBETTER DH, Isolation of anonymous DNA sequences from within a submicroscopic X chromosomal deletion in a patient with choroideremia, deafness, and mental retardation. Proc Nati Acad Sci USA, 84, 6521-6525., 1987.

20 -   ROPERS HH, ZUFFARDI O, BIANCHI E, TIEPOLO L, Agenesis of corpus callosum, ocular and skeletal anomalies (X-linked dominant Aicardi's Syndrome) in a girl with balanced X/3 translocation. Human Genet, 61, 364-368., 1982.

21 -   ROSENBERG T, SCHWARTZ M, NEIBUHR E, YANNG HM, SARDEMANN H, ANDERSEN O, LUNDSTEEN C, Choroideremia in interstitial deletion of the X chromosome. Ophtalmic Paediatr Genet, 7, 205-210., 1986.

22 -   SCHWARTZ M, ROSENBERG T, NIEBUHR E, LUNDSTEEN C, SARDEMANN H, ANDERSEN O, YANG HM, LAMM LU, Choroideremia : further evidence for assgnement of the locus to Xq13-Xq21. Hum Genet, 74, 449-452., 1986.

23 -   SEFIANI A, SINNETT D, ABEL L, SZPIRO-TAPIA S, HEUERTZ S, CRAIG I, FRASER N, KRUSE TA, FRYDMAN M, PETER MO, SCHMUTZ JL, GILGENKRANTZ S, MITTCHELL G, FREZAL J, MELANCON S, LAVERGNE, LABUDA D, HORS-CAYLA MC, Linkage studies do not confirm the cytogenetic location of incontinentia pigmenti on Xp11. Hum Genet, 80, 282-286., 1988

24 -   SIU VM, GONDER JR, SERGOVICH FR, FLINTOFF WF, Choroideremia associated with an X-autosomal translocation. J Hum Genet, 43, n°359 (abstract), 1988.

25 -   VERELLEN-DUMOULIN C, FREUND M, DEMEYER R, LATERRE, FREDERIC J, THOMPSON MW, MARKOVIC VD, WORTON R, Expression of an X-linked muscular dystrophy in a female due to non-random inactivation of the normal X-chromosome. Hum Genet 67, 115-119., 1984.

26 -   ZONANA J, CLARKE A, SARFARAZI M, THOMAS NST, ROBERTS K, MARYMEE K, HARPER PS, X-linked hypohidrotic ectodermal dysplasia : localization within the region Xq11-21.1 by linkage analysis and implications for carrier detection and prenatal diagnosis. Am J Hum Genet, 43, 75-85., 1988.

ABSTRACT

DE NOVO BALANCED (X;7) TRANSLOCATION ASSOCIATED WITH CHOROIDEREMIA AND PRIMARY AMENORRHEA ; A STUDY OF THE Xq21.2 BREAKPOINT.

A 24 year-old woman with choroideremia and primary amenorrhea was found to have a de novo translocation with breakpoint at Xq21.2. GTG, QFQ and RBA bandings showed the chromosome constitution : 46,X, t(X;7) (q21.2;p14) and the non-random inactivation of normal X. We suggest that the breakpoint occured in choroideremia gene and also in the critical region responsible for gonadal dysgenesis. Molecular studies of the breakpoint from somatic cell hybrid may contribute to define this region.

MOLECULAR GENETIC STUDIES IN AUTOSOMAL DOMINANT RETINITIS PIGMENTOSA

R Bashir[1], CF Inglehearn[1], D Lester[1],
B Lauffart[1], J Keen[1], SS Papiha[1],
M Jay[2], AC Bird[2] and SS Bhattacharya[1]

INTRODUCTION

The molecular genetics of autosomal dominant retinitis pigmentosa (ADRP) has made remarkable progress since the first reported linkage of one form of ADRP to the long arm of chromosome 3[1]. In a large Irish pedigree named TCDM1, with type1 ADRP, the disease was found to be strongly linked to the 3q marker C17 (D3S47) with a lod score of +14.7 at zero recombination, indicating that C17 was very close if not in the ADRP gene itself. Since this linkage report we have been studying the ADRP families on our genetic register and this chapter details the findings to date.

LINKAGE STUDIES WITH C17 (D3S47)

Following the linkage report by McWilliam et al[1], our laboratory was the first to demonstrate genetic heterogeneity in ADRP[2]. This was shown in a large ADRP family called AD5 (Figure 1) which is clinically distinct from TCDM1 in terms of age of onset and loss of photoreceptor function. Negative linkage was recorded between ADRP and C17 (lod score of -2 at 10% recombination). Clinical heterogeneity in ADRP had long been established with classification into type I or D type and type II or R type, corresponding to diffuse and regional loss of photoreceptor function respectively[3,4]. Onset of blindness is relatively early in life in type I or D type and relatively mixed in type II or R type. Figure 1 shows further two large ADRP families, AD3, classified clinically as type I or D type and AD7 classified as type II or R type. Linkage data for these families and others is summarized in Table 1 which also includes the data for TCDMI [1] and the results of Ollsson et al[5].

1 Molecular Genetics Unit, University of Newcastle-upon Tyne, UK
2 Moorfields Eye Hospital, London, UK

ADRP 5

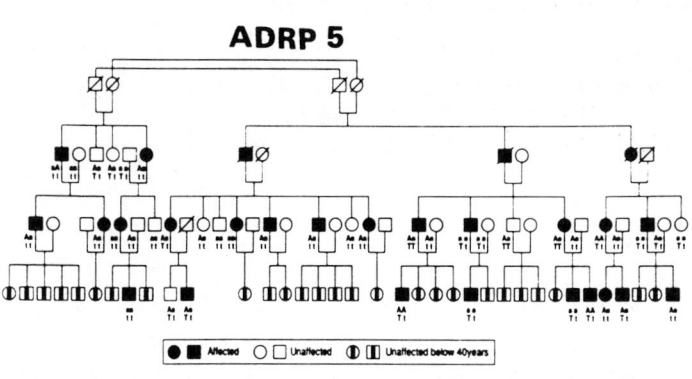

ADRP3 (D)

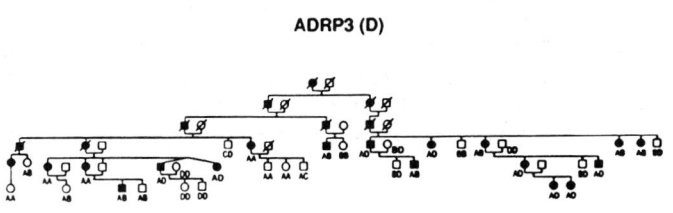

ADRP7 (R)

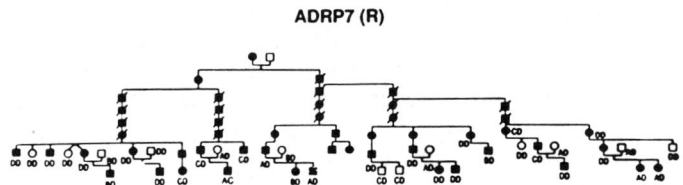

Figure 1
Pedigrees of three of our large ADRP families in our ADRP register.
In ADRP 5 and 7, clinically classified as R type or Type II with incomplete penetrance no linkage between ADRP and C17 is observed.
In ADRP 3, clinically classified as D type or Type I, the disease is linked to C17.

AD3 and AD14 both classified as type I or D type like TCDM1 show linkage to C17 at zero recombination; in family 20 an Australian pedigree as reported in Ollsson et al[5], linkage between ADRP and C17 is seen at 8% recombination indicating the possibility of another ADRP locus on 3q near C17. AD5 and AD7 both classified as type II or R type with incomplete penetrance show no linkage to C17[1,6].

TABLE 1
Linkage data of C17 v ADRP

ADRP FAMILY (D or R)	RECOMBINATION FRACTION θ						
	0.00	0.01	0.05	0.10	0.20	0.30	0.40
AD3 (D)	+5.61	+5.60	+5.39	+4.96	+3.86	+2.58	+1.17
AD14 (D)	+2.69	+2.67	+2.42	+2.12	+1.48	+0.81	+0.25
TCDM (D)	+14.7	+14.0	+13.54	+12.32	+9.68	+6.72	+3.38
FAMILY 20 (R)	− ∞	+3.05	+4.59	+4.78	+4.14	+2.98	+1.55
AD5 (R)	− ∞	−10.6	−5.28	−3.15	−1.27	−0.44	−0.07
AD7 (R)	− ∞	−4.12	−2.02	−1.18	−0.49	−0.21	−0.08

RHODOPSIN

Rhodopsin an integral membrane protein found in the rod outer segment (ROS) has an essential role in the complex phototransduction cascade. Its vital role in vision and location on 3q[7] near C17 immediately made it the primary candidate gene for ADRP families showing linkage to C17. The gene for this protein had been cloned and sequenced by Nathans et al[8] therefore it was not difficult to determine if there was a mutation in this gene in the affected individuals in these families. A few months after the linkage report of McWilliam et al[1], Dryja et al[9] were the first to demonstrate a point mutation in the first exon in codon 23 of the rhodopsin gene in 17 out of 148 unrelated patients with ADRP and in none of the 102 normals. The C to A transversion in codon 23 changed the amino acid sequence from proline to histidine. By direct genomic sequencing to PCR amplified first exon and hybridisation of kinase end labelled oligomers spanning the 23rd codon and corresponding to the normal and mutant sequences, we were unable to detect this mutation in AD3, one of our C17 linked families[6]. Figure II shows the dot blot of normals and affected patients from AD3 hybridised with the normal and the mutant oligomers, the normal oligomer gives a strong hybridisation signal in both normals and affecteds whereas the mutant oligomer displays a weak signal in both. These results were further confirmed by direct genomic sequencing (Figure III), both normals and affecteds from AD3 have the sequence GGG at the 23rd codon when the gel is read from 3'terminus to 5'. By oligo dot blot hybridisation we were

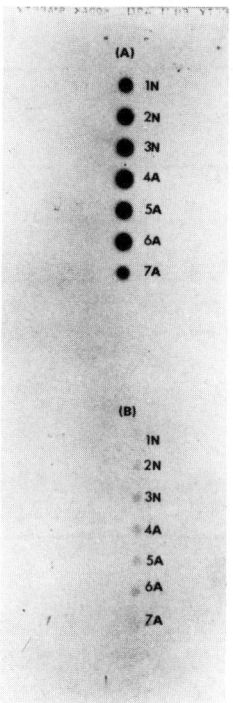

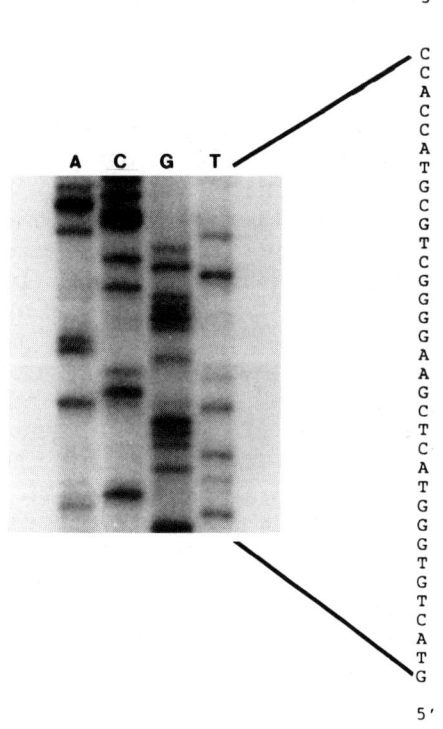

Figure II(left)
Dot blot of PCR amplified exon 1 of normals (1N→3N) and affecteds (4A→7A) from ADRP3 hybridised with (A) the normal oligomer and (B) the mutant oligomer. The normal oligomer hybridises strongly to normals and affecteds in contrast to the mutant oligomer which gives a weak signal indicating the abscence of the codon 23 mutation in this C17 linked family.

Figure III (right)
Sequence analysis of an affected from ADRP3 showing a normal rhodopsin sequence at and around the 23 codon. Rhodopsin 1st exon DNA was amplified and then primed with the internal oligomer 5'GCTAGGTTGAGCAGGATGTA3'

unable to detect this point mutation in a further 25 unrelated ADRP families[10]. To date the data from our laboratory and from those of Pete Humphries and A. Gal confirm the abscence of this mutation in 90 unrelated ADRP families[11] indicating this mutation to be very rare in Europe[11]. How a mutation at the 23rd codon causes ADRP is as yet unknown.

Rhodopsin is arranged as seven transmembrane helices, the amino terminal is intradiskal and the carboxy terminal is cytoplasmic[12]. Most of the interactions between rhodopsin and other proteins involved in phototransduction occurr at the cytoplasmic surface and not at the amino terminal near codon 23. However, the proline at codon 23 is highly conserved in opsins from Drosophila to human and other proteins like the B-adrenergic receptor[12] and the conversion of a highly conserved proline to a charged histidine may therefore alter the secondary structure and hence the stability of the molecule in the rod outer segment. Since the codon 23 mutation was not responsible for ADRP in any of our C17 linked families, we had to ascertain (i) if rhodopsin is the ADRP gene in these families and (ii) identify the mutations within. The possibility of another ADRP locus also existed but before pursuing this we had to investigate points (i) and (ii). The rhodopsin gene is not very large (4-5kb) and is divided into five exons. We synthesised primers to the entire gene at the intron-exon boundaries as well as internal primers to each exon and continued to study rhodopsin by a) direct genomic sequencing and b) linkage analysis using the microsatellite repeat in exon 1[13] and flanking DNA markers around rhodopsin and C17[14]. Direct genomic sequencing proved to be the most fruitful and in one C17 linked family, AD14, we were able to identify a three base pair deletion in exon IV of the rhodopsin gene (Figure IV) resulting in the removal of an isoleucine residue at codon 255 or 256[10].

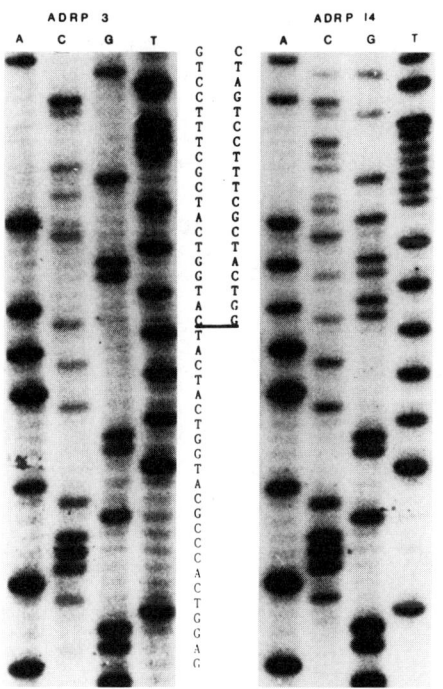

Figure IV
Sequence analysis at exon IV of an affected from AD3 and AD14. Comparison of the sequence data indicates the presence of a three base pair deletion in AD14 at codon 255/256.

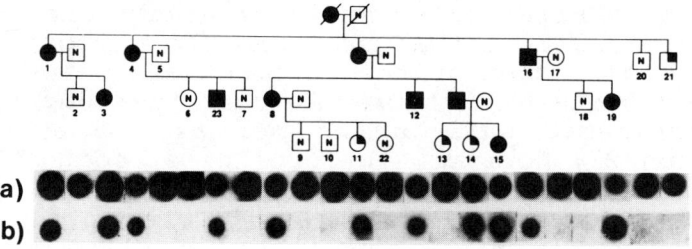

<u>Figure V</u>   Oligo dot hybridisation to PCR amplified
rhodopsin fourth exon in AD14. a) represents
the hybridisation signal with the normal
oligomer and b) the mutant oligomer. The three
base pair deletion at exon IV segregates with
ADRP in this family indicating it to be the
causative defect.

By synthesising oligomers spanning the normal and deleted
region and oligo-dot hybridisation to PCR amplified
fourth exon we were able to confirm the presence of this
mutation and its segregation with ADRP in this family
(Figure V). PCR amplification of a 100bp fragment within
this region could also be resolved on a 10%
polyacrylamide gel, unaffecteds appearing a a single band
of 100bp, reflecting two copies of normal rhodopsin
sequence, while affecteds show two bands of 100bp and 97
bp respectively (Figure VI). Also this deletion and
others were tested in exon IV from 30 other unrelated
families, with ADRP and other retinal disorders and found
to be absent[10]. Unlike codon 23, codon 255 or 256 are not
conserved in opsins but found in proteins like
rhodopsin and B-adrenergic receptor[12]. Which isoleucine
residue is deleted is not known but a consequence of the
deletion would be a shortening of the sixth transmembrane
helical domain altering the secondary structure of the
molecule.
Interestingly, the isoleucine residue deleted is in a run
of three TCA repeats and one can postulate a mechanism by
which this deletion has arisen; replication slippage at
meiosis is a mechanism thought to be significant in the
formation of short tandem repeats at microsatellite loci

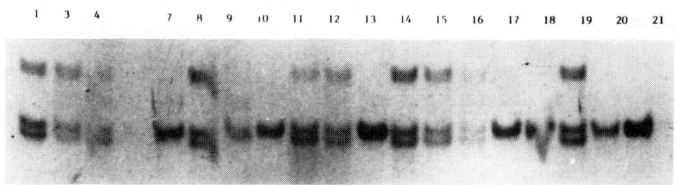

Figure VI   Polyacrylamide gel electrophoresis of a 100 bp
             PCR amplified fragment in AD14, normals
             appearing as a single band of 100 bp and
             affecteds as three bands, two representing the
             normal and deleted rhodopsin fragments
             respectively and the upper band corresponding
             to heteroduplexes of normal and deleted
             fragments formed in the PCR reaction.

although unequal crossing over might also be a possible
cause[14]. If these mechanisms are significant in the
production of such deletions, it would appear that coding
seqences are not exempt from these processes.
Thus the clinical heterogeneity in ADRP reflected at the
genetic level is also present at the molecular level.
There is more than one locus for ADRP, possible two on 3q
and at least four different mutations to date within
rhodopsin, codon 23, 58, and 347 all identified by Dryja
et al[9,16] and codon 255 or 256 as discussed in this
chapter and in Inglehearn et al[10]. Other proteins
involved in the phototransduction cascade are now also
candidate genes for other forms of ADRP. Identification
of such genes and mutations will provide predictive
testing and counselling in ADRP families. Research aimed
at elucidating the pathophysiology of these mutations in
ADRP has also begun with the use of transgenic mice
incorporating such mutations as the one at codon 23[16].
Such experiments will provide valuable insights to the
etiology of this disease and hence possible therapy at
the genetic and/or pharmacological levels.

REFERENCES

1. McWilliam,P., Farrar, G.J., Kenna, P., Bradley, D.J., Marian, M.M., Sharp E.M., McConnel, D.J., Lawler, M., Shiels, D., Ryan, C., Stevens, K., Daiger, S.P. and Humphries, P., Autosomal dominant retinitis pigmentosa (ADRP): Localization of an ADRP gene to the long arm of chromosome 3, <u>Genomics</u> 5, 619, 1989.

2. Inglehearn, C.F., Jay, M., Lester, D., Bashir, R., Jay, B., Bird, A.C., Wright , A.F., Evans, H.J., Papiha, S.S. and Bhattacharya, S.S, No evidence for linkage between late onset autosomal retinitis pigmentosa and chromosome 3 locus D3S47 (C17): Evidence for genetic heterogeneity, <u>Genomics</u> 6, 168, 1990.

3. Massof, R.W. and Finkelstein, D.C., Two forms of autosomal dominant retinitis pigmentosa, <u>Doc. Ophthalmol.</u> 51, 289,1971.

4. Arden, G.B., Carter, R.M., Hogg, C.G., Powell, D.J., Ernst, W.J.K., Clover, G.M., Lyness, A.AL, Quinlan, M.P., Rod and cone activity in patients with dominantly inherited retinitis pigmentosa: comparisons between psychophysical and electroretinotgraphic measurements, <u>Brit. J. Ophthalmol.</u> 67, 405, 1983.

5. Ollsson, J.E., Samanns, C., Jeminez, J., Pongratz, J., Chand, A., Watly, A., Seuchter, S.A., Denton, M. and Gal, A., Gene for Type II autosomal dominant retinitis pigmentosa maps on the long arm of chromosome 3, <u>Am. J. Med. Genet.</u>, 35.595,1990.

6. Lester, D.H., Inglehearn, C.F., Bashir, R., Ackfor, I.H., Eskowitz, L., Jay, M., Bird, A.C., Wright, A.T. and Bhattacharya, S.S. (1990), Linkage to D3547 (C17) in one large family and exclusion in another: confirmation of genetic heterogeneity. <u>Am. J. Hum. Genet.</u>, 47, 536, 1990.

7. Human Gene Mapping 10

8. Nathans, J. and Hogness, D.S., Isolation and nucleotide sequencing of the gene encoding human rhodopsin, <u>PNAS. USA.</u> 81, 4851, 1983.

9. Dryja, T.P., McGee, T.L., Reichel, E., Hahu, L.B., Cowley, G.S., Yandell, D.W., Sandberg, M.A. and Berson, E.L., A point mutation of the rhodopsin gene in one form of RP, <u>Nature</u> 343, 364, 1990.

10. Inglehearn, C.F., Bashir, R., Lester, D.H., Jay, M., Bird, A.C. and Bhattacharya S.S., A three base pair deletion in the rhodopsin gene in a family with autosomal dominant retinitis pigmantosa, _Am. J. Hum. Genet._ 47, 536, 1990.

11. Farrar, G.J., Kenna P., Redmond, R., McWilliam, P., Bradley, D.G., Humphries, M.M., Sharp, E.M., Inglehearn, C.F., Bashir, R., Jay, M., Watty, A., Ludwig, M., Schinzel, A., Samanns, C., Gal, A., Bhattacharya, S.S. and Humphries, P., Autosamal dominant retinitis pigmentosa: Abscence of the rhodopsin codon 23 proline histidine substitution in pedigrees of Irish origin, _Am. J. Hum. Genet._ 47, 1990.

12. Applebury, M.L. and Hargrave P.A.C., Molecular biology of the visual pigments, _Vis. Res._ 26, 1881, 1986.

13. Weber, T.L. and May, P.E.., Abundant class of human DNA polymorphisms which can be typed using the polymerase chain reaction, _Am. J. Hum. Genet._ 44, 388, 1989.

14. Donis-Keller et al, A genetic linkage map of the human genome, _Cell_, 51,319,1987.

15. Jarman, P.J. and Wells, R.A., Hypervariable minisatellites: recombinators or innocent bystanders? _Trends in Genet._ 5, 367,1989.

16. Ollsson, J. et al, IRPA Meeting, Dublin, 1990.

LINKAGE MAPPING AND MOLECULAR STUDIES OF AUTOSOMAL FORMS OF RETINITIS PIGMENTOSA

Stephen P. Daiger*, Susan H. Blanton*, Anne Cottingham*, Jana Laidlaw*, Joseph A. Rodriguez*, John R. Heckenlively†

*Medical Genetics Center, The University of Texas Health Science Center, Houston, Texas, USA; †Jules Stein Eye Institute, University of California, Los Angeles, California, USA

I. INTRODUCTION

For the past six years our research in Houston has focused on linkage mapping and, more recently, on molecular studies of autosomal forms of retinitis pigmentosa (RP). The principal diseases we have studied are autosomal dominant retinitis pigmentosa (ADRP) and Usher syndrome (US). We have worked as part of a collaborative network known as the Support Program for DNA Linkage Studies of Degenerative Retinal Diseases, funded by the National Retinitis Pigmentosa Foundation, Inc., the George Gund Foundation and the National Institutes of Health.[1] Goals of the Support Program include 1.) identification and clinical characterization of families suitable for DNA linkage studies, 2.) collection of blood samples for preparation and storage of transformed cell lines by the Human Genetic Mutant Cell Repository, Camden, New Jersey, USA, and 3.) linkage and molecular studies in collaboration with other investigators.

Primary collaborators, their institutions and their roles include the following:
* John R. Heckenlively, MD; Jules Stein Eye Institute, Univ. of California, Los Angeles, California, USA -- ascertainment and clinical evaluation of families and patients with ADRP;
* Mary Z. Pelias, PhD; Dept. of Biometry and Genetics, Louisiana State Univ. Medical School, New Orleans, Louisiana, USA -- ascertainment and clinical evaluation of families with US;
* J. Fielding Hejtmancik, MD, PhD, and Richard A. Smith, MD; Institute for Molecular Genetics, Baylor College of Medicine, Houston, Texas, USA -- clinical evaluation and laboratory investigation of families with US;
* Charles A. Garcia, MD; Herman Eye Center, The Univ. of Texas Health Science Center, Houston; and Richard A. Lewis, MD; Cullen Eye Institute, Baylor College of Medicine -- ascertainment and clinical evaluation of families and patients with ADRP;
* Robert A. Sparkes, MD, PhD, and M. Anne Spence, PhD; Univ. of California, Los Angeles -- laboratory investigation and computational analysis of families with ADRP; and
* Peter Humphries, PhD; Dept. of Genetics, Trinity College Dublin, Ireland -- laboratory investigation of families with ADRP.

II. FAMILIES

To date, blood samples from members of two extended families have been submitted to the Cell Repository. The families are 1.) UCLA-RP01, an eight-generation family with late-onset, type II ADRP,[2] and 2.) LSU-US01, a collection of genetically-related nuclear families with type II US.[3] UCLA-RP01 is an American family, of Western European origin, located in Kentucky, USA; it has been the subject of extensive studies by Dr. Heckenlively and his colleagues over a number of years.[2,4-6] LSU-US01 is a set of nuclear families, with large sibships, of French-Acadian descent living in southwestern Louisiana, USA. US families in this geographically isolated population share common ancestors in the 18th century. LSU-US01 has been the subject of extensive studies by Dr. Pelias and her colleagues.[3,7-11] Dr. Pelias reports further on these families, and on related linkage studies, in another manuscript in this volume.[12]

Currently the RP Cell Line Collection in the Cell Repository has 136 cell lines from UCLA-RP01 and 91 cell lines from LSU-US01 (Table 1).[13,14] These cell lines are available to the scientific community for linkage studies and other investigations. In addition, we have submitted blood samples from a nuclear family (an affected mother, unaffected father and affected son) with the codon 23 mutation in rhodopsin.[15] Cell lines from the latter family, UTAD-010, should be available shortly.

TABLE 1

Cell Lines in the RP Cell Line Collection in the Human Genetic Mutant
Cell Repository, Camden, New Jersey, USA

Family	Total Samples Submitted	Total Individuals Submitted	Total Transformed	Total DNAs
UCLA-RP01	166	143	136	136
LSU-US01	102	95	91	81
UTAD-010	3	3	3	3

III. LINKAGE STUDIES of UCLA-RP01

A. EFFECTIVENESS of UCLA-RP01 for LINKAGE ANALYSIS.

The UCLA-RP01 pedigree (Figure 1) is typical of many families used for linkage studies of dominant diseases: numerous affected individuals are known but the number of living, available individuals is substantially less than the total number required for computation of linkage scores. DNAs and blood samples are available from all living family members shown in Figure 1 but several individuals are missing from the grandparental generation, there are no living great grandparents and individuals in the most recent generation are often separated from each other by 6 generations, that is, by 12 meiotic events. Also, in this particular family, there are two inbreeding loops which profoundly increase the time for linkage calculations.

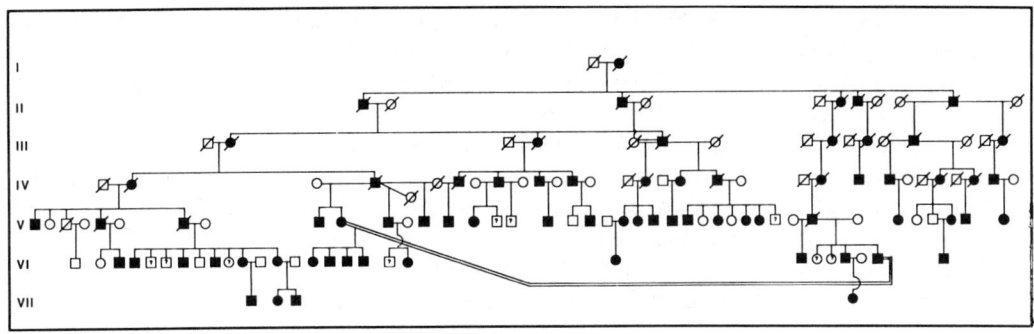

Figure 1. Pedigree of ADRP family UCLA-RP01.

(In one nuclear family in Figure 1, two parents who share a common, affected ancestor are themselves affected. Two children of these affected parents are severely affected with early-onset disease, while the onset in other family members is typically age 20-30 years and symptoms are usually mild. These two individuals may be homozygous for the disease gene, suggesting that in this form of ADRP, having two copies of the RP gene is worse than having one. This is in contrast to Huntington disease where the homozygous state is not clinically different from the heterozygous state.[16] These homozygous RP individuals may be of assistance in isolating the disease gene subsequent to linkage mapping.)

The consequences of these characteristics of the UCLA-RP01 pedigree are that linkage testing is computationally slow and that the log odds (LOD) scores are unusually sensitive to the choice of allele frequencies.[17,18] Also, as is true for all linkage studies but is particularly important in this instance, accurate diagnosis and incorporation of a conservative age-of-onset correction are essential. We have dealt with these potential difficulties in several ways. First, we have made numerous field trips to visit family members and to collect blood samples from as many appropriate individuals as possible. All blood samples are transformed; where transformation is unsuccessful, as is occasionally the case, unfortunately, for samples from elderly blood donors, skin fibroblasts are prepared. Second, if the diagnostic classification of an at-risk individual is equivocal, then the individual is either not included in the study or is given an extended retinal examination at the Jules Stein Eye Institute, Los Angeles, or at a similar facility. Third, our linkage computations, using either the computer program LIPED[19] for two-point analysis or LINKAGE[20] for multipoint calculations, incorporates the following age-of-onset correction for at-risk, apparently unaffected individuals: those under 30 are entered as "unknown", those 30 to 39 are given a 20% chance of possessing an unexpressed ADRP gene, those 40 to 49 are given a 10% chance, and those over 50 are scored as "unaffected".[2] This conservative approach may bias our calculations against detection of linkage but it should also substantially reduce the false positive rate.

Further responses to problems with linkage analysis include, fourth, attempts to use very high speed computational methods[16] and, fifth, splitting the family into smaller, more manageable blocks to simplify calculations. Though neither of these approaches has proven completely satisfactory, a combination of "quick", two-point calculations on the split family followed by slow (*very* slow!) multipoint calculations on the entire family has been sufficient so far. However, development of enhanced methods for linkage computations continues to be one of our major goals.

In spite of these potential difficulties, UCLA-RP01 is demonstrably satisfactory for effective linkage testing using DNA markers. Computer simulation of the results of linkage testing in UCLA-RP01, using the computer program SIMLINK,[21] demonstrates that this family is as informative as was the first ADRP family within which linkage was detected, TCD-M[22] (Table 2). As an example, at a genetic distance of 5cM (centiMorgans) a typical marker would produce a LOD score of over 3 in 94% of cases in UCLA-RP01. Thus we are confident that when, eventually, the correct marker is tested, unequivocal linkage to ADRP in UCLA-RP01 will be detected.

TABLE 2

SIMLINK Results: Power to Include or Exclude Linkage in
UCLA-RP01 and TCD-M Using a Three-Allele Marker System

A. Inclusion: probability of LOD score ≥ 3.0

Average θ	Average prob. in UCLA-RP01	Average prob. in TCDM-1
0.00	1.00	0.98
0.05	0.94	0.92
0.10	0.75	0.82
0.15	0.53	0.55

B. Exclusion: probability of LOD score ≤ -2.0

Test θ	Average prob. in UCLA-RP01	Average prob. in TCDM-1
0.00	1.00	0.99
0.05	0.99	0.96
0.10	0.87	0.85
0.20	0.37	0.40

B. SELECTION of LINKAGE MARKERS in UCLA-RP01.

Obvious goals in selecting markers for linkage testing are to select markers which are 1.) sufficiently informative, 2.) easily and unequivocally typed and 3.) optimally spaced so that multipoint linkage methods may be used. Where feasible we have selected markers which flank previously tested markers or which complete linkage groups spanning whole chromosomes or chromosome regions. In spite of the advantage in analyzing linkage groups, though, we have found that it is usually more efficient to select easily-tested markers scattered throughout the genome than to select markers to completely exclude specific chromosome regions.

Regarding useful markers, the potentially most informative markers, VNTRs (variable number of tandem repeats),[23] with very high heterozygosity, are not useful, unfortunately, in large, sparse pedigrees such as UCLA-RP01. This is because of the difficulty in distinguishing alleles of similar molecular weight when not all parents are tested. Additionally, VNTR allele frequencies are uncertain in most cases.

Our most useful markers have turned out to be simple restriction-site polymorphisms where a single probe can detect more than one RFLP (restriction fragment length polymorphism) site. Such markers are easily tested, the resulting types are unambiguous and, by constructing haplotypes, the systems can be highly informative. Also, allele frequencies are usually known and haplotype frequencies are easily calculated, assuming linkage equilibrium. Examples of such marker systems are shown in Table 3.

TABLE 3
Loci Tested for Linkage to ADRP in UCLA-RP01

Symbol	Chromosome	Symbol	Chromosome
PND*	1p36	D4S118	4q
ALPL*	1p36.1-p34	BF	6p21.3
RH	1p36.2-p34	DQβ	6p21.3
D1S57	1pter-p31	GLO1	6p21.3-p21.1
PGM1	1p22.1	CF*	7q31-q32
AMY	1p21	D8S26	8q22-q23
FY	1q21-q25	D8S39	8
D2S1*	2p25	GPT	8q23-qter
ACP1	2p25	ASS*	9q11-q22
APOB	2p24-23	ABO	9q34.1-q34.2
D2S3	2q35-37	RBP3	10q11.2
TF	3q21	TYR	11q14-q12
D3S47*	3q21-q22	ESD	13q14.1-14.2
D3S14	3q21-q22	RB1	13q14.2
D3S32	3cen	PI	14q32.1
D4S10	4p16.3-p16.2	PGP	16p13
D4S23	4p16.1 or p15.1	HP	16q22
D4S40	4q21-qter	D17S30	17
D4S21	4p16.1 or p15.1	INSR	19p13.3-p1
D4S18	4p16.1-p15.1	LE	19p13.3-p1
D4S44	4q11-qter	C3	19p13.3-p1
D4S16	4p15.1-q11	APOC1	19q12-q13.2
GC	4q12-q13	D21S58	21q21
MNS	4q28-31	P1	22q11.2-qter

*DNA locus with more than one polymorphic site.

Finally, the most promising development in DNA linkage testing recently has been the application of methods based on the polymerase chain reaction (PCR)[24] to detection of polymorphic variation. To date we have tested over 10 PCR-detectable polymorphisms in UCLA-RP01 (Table 4).[25-27] These include several loci with more than one restriction site variant and one candidate gene locus, retinol binding protein 3 (RBP3) on the short arm of chromosome 10.[28] In our experience testing "PCR polymorphisms" requires about one-third the time required by Southern gel analysis and is substantially less prone to artifacts.

TABLE 4
Polymorphisms Tested Using PCR Amplification

Gene	Map Location		Primers	Polym[*]
Apolipoprotein B	2p24-p23		5'-ATGGAAACGGAGAAATTATG-3' 5'-CCTTCTCACTTGGCAAATAC-3'	VNTR
Apoliprotein C1	19qter		5'-TTTGAGCTCGGCTCTTGAGACAGGAA-3' 5'-GGTCCCGGGCACTTCCCTTAGCCCCA-3'	RS
Cystic fibrosis	7q31	a.	5'-GTTGAAGTGAATTGAATG-3' 5'-TGAGTCTCTGCTGCCAGT-3'	RS
		b.	5'-CCACTGATACTGTGAGAC-3' 5'-GTTGTTTCAAGTCACTGC-3'	
D17S30	17		5'-CGAAGAGTGAAGTGCACAGG -3' 5'-CACAGTCTTTATTCTTCAGCG-3'	VNTR
Insulin receptor	19p13.3-p13.2		5'-GAATTCACATTCCCAAGACA-3' 5'-CGGTCTTGTAAGGGTAACTG-3'	RS
Rhodopsin	3q21-qter		5'-CACAGAAGGCCCTAACTTCT-3' 5'-GCACGATCAGCAGAAACATG-3'	Dis.
Rhodopsin	3q21-qter		5'-CATTAGGATGCATTCTTCTG-3' 5'-GTCAGGATTGAACTGGGAAC-3	CA
Retinoblastoma susceptibility locus	13q14		5'-TTCCAATGAAGAACAAATGG-3' 5'-GCAATTGCACAATCCAAGTT-3'	RS
Retinol-binding protein (RBP3)	10p11.2-q11.2		5'-CATTCCTGGAATTGTGCCCA-3' 5'-CAAATACTTCAGGGGAAGGG-3'	RS
Tyrosinase	11q14-q12		5'-GCAAGTTTGGCTTTTGGGGA-3' 5'-CTGCCAAGAGGAGAAGAATG-3'	RS

[*]Polymorphism type: VNTR = variable number of tandem repeats; RS = restriction site; Dis. = disease mutation; CA = microsatellite CA repeat.

C. LINKAGE RESULTS with UCLA-RP01.

Tables 3 and 4 summarize all polymorphic loci tested for linkage to the ADRP locus in UCLA-RP01. In earlier studies linkage between ADRP and the Rh blood group, at chromosome location 1q34, was suggested by studies in this family.[6] However, multipoint linkage testing using the linkage group PND - ALPA - Rh - D1S57 - PGM1, clearly excludes the locus from this region in the family.[29,30] Also, multipoint analysis excludes the disease locus from most of chromosome 4.[2] Further, and most importantly, the ADRP locus in UCLA-RP01 can be excluded from ± 17cM around D3S47, the locus which shows tight linkage to other forms of ADRP and to rhodopsin.[22,31] Thus the ADRP locus in this family is genetically distinct from the locus in 3q-linked families and provides additional evidence of genetic heterogeneity in autosomal dominant retinitis pigmentosa.

In summary, we have tested over 48 markers in UCLA-RP01 and have excluded the locus from over one-third of the human genome.[32] An approximate exclusion map can be generated using the computer program EXCLUDE,[33] as shown in Figure 4. EXCLUDE assigns an *a priori* probability of linkage to each human chromosome based on its relative length and then adjusts these probabilities based on linkage data. In Figure 4 the height of each chromosomal box is proportional to the length of the chromosome but its area is proportional to the adjusted, *a posteriori* probability of linkage. Thus, as an example, the relative area (shown to the right of the chromosome number) of chromosome 4 is 0.0 since this chromosome has been excluded. When linkage is still possible, on chromosome 2 as an example, the black curve indicates the likelihood of each location. Please note, though, that although this is a useful device for displaying all accumulated linkage results in this family, the probabilities are approximations at best.

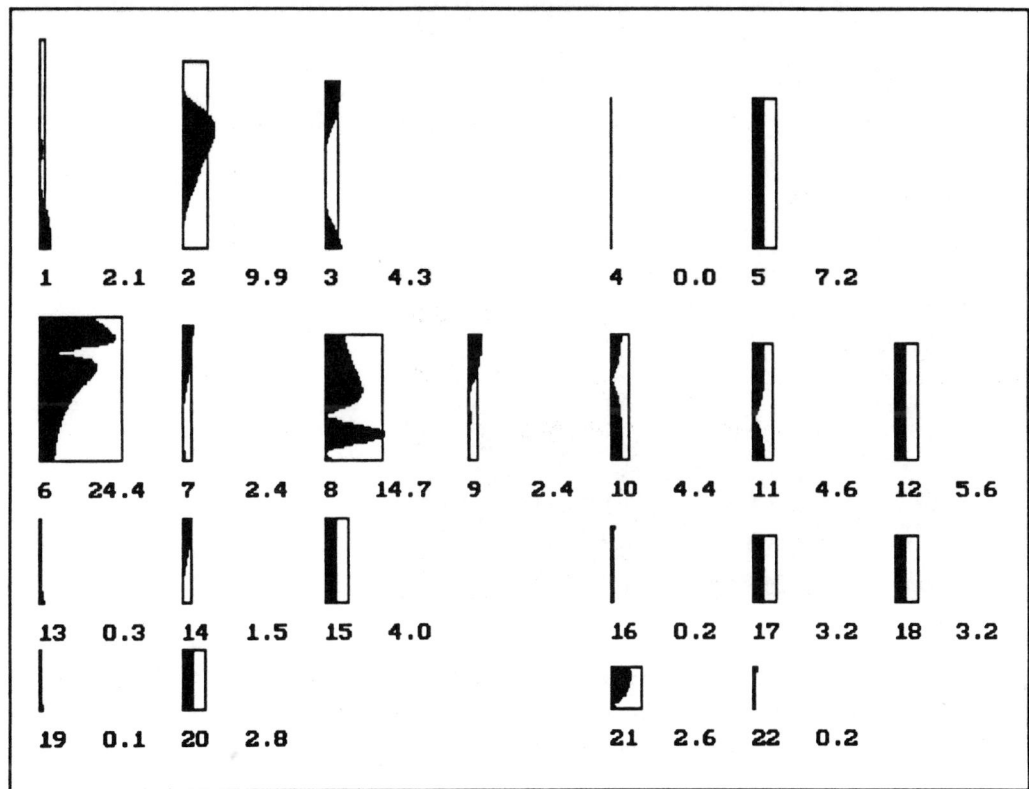

Figure 2. Exclusion map of the ADRP locus in UCLA-RP01.

IV. TESTING for CODON 23 MUTATIONS in ADRP FAMILIES and PATIENTS

Following the report by Dryja et al. of a mutation at codon 23 (exon 1) of rhodopsin as the cause of ADRP in approximately 15% of American families[34], we began to collect and test genomic DNA samples from unrelated, Caucasian families with apparent autosomal dominant retinitis pigmentosa.   To test for the codon 23 mutation we selected two 20-nucleotide primers which amplify a 140bp (base pair) segment of exon 1 of rhodopsin (Table 4 and Figure 3). The codon 23 site is roughly in the center of this sequence. We then selected two 15bp probes, one specific to the mutant sequence and the other specific to the wild-type sequence, and tested for the mutation using allele specific oligonucleotide (ASO) hybridization (Figure 4).[15,35]

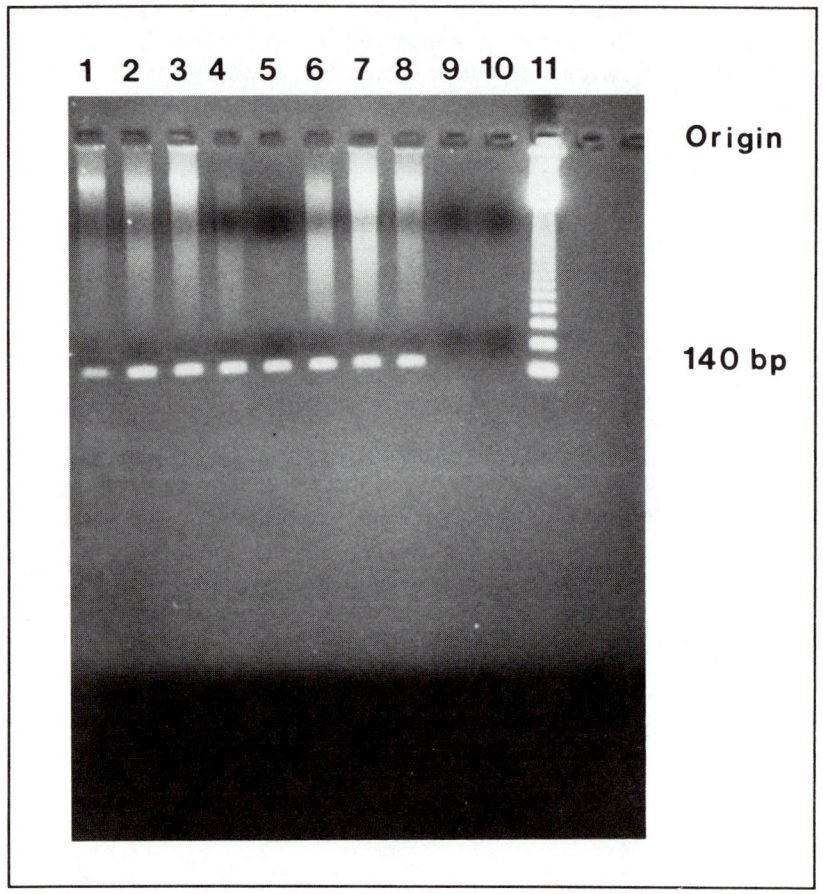

Figure 3. PCR amplification of rhodopsin exon 1 in human genomic DNA. Lanes 1-8: DNAs from unrelated humans; lanes 9-10: blank controls; lane 11: 123bp (base pair) ladder for molecular weight determination.

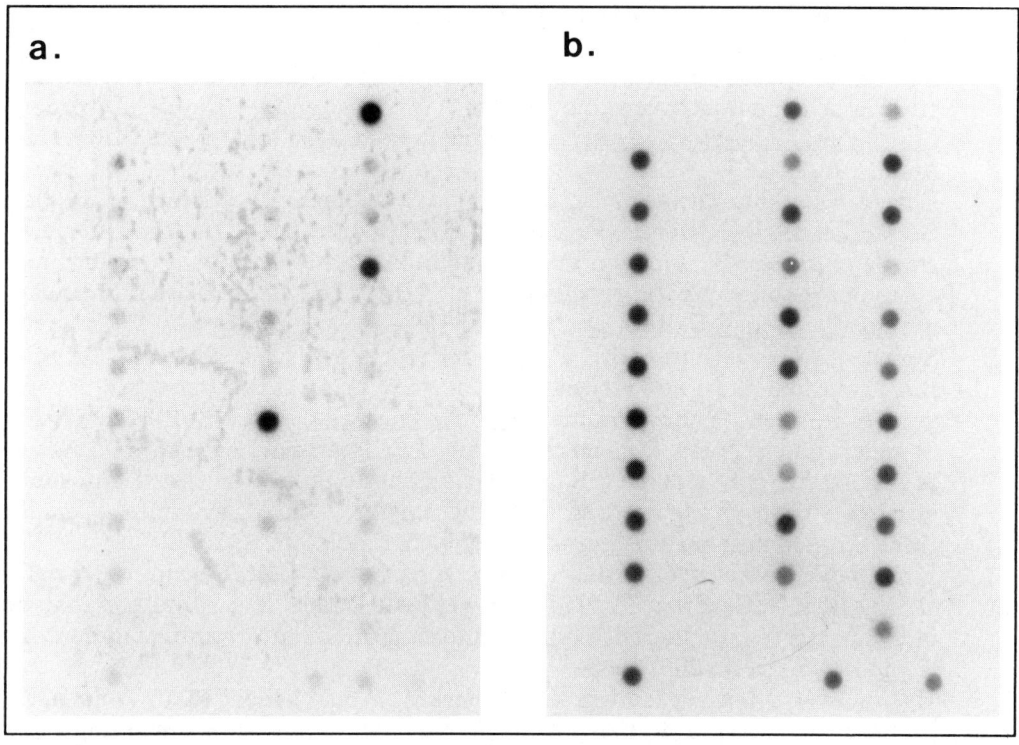

Figure 4. ASO detection of rhodopsin codon 23. a: mutant ASO (for codon 23); b: wilt-type ASO.

Within the first 14 samples tested, we observed two positive individuals. In both cases the affected parent of the proband also carried the codon 23 mutation thus confirming Mendelian inheritance. What was most unusual about these two families was that both have "sectoral RP"[36], which is characterized by asymmetric involvement between upper and lower visual fields, or segmental retinal degenerative changes, often leaving demarcation lines between normal-appearing posterior pole and atrophied inferior equatorial retina. (Additional details are reported elsewhere.[15])

Whether the codon 23 mutation or other specific mutations will predominate among sectoral RP families, or even whether all sectoral cases will involve an alteration in rhodopsin, will require further research. In any case, this finding illustrates the profound clinical insights which are certain to emerge from the developing molecular understanding of degenerative retinal diseases.

ACKNOWLEDGEMENTS. This research was supported by grants from the National Retinitis Pigmentosa Foundation, Inc., USA, and the George Gund Foundation, by Grant Number EY07142 from the National Institutes of Health and by a grant from the John J. Roscia Family.

VI. REFERENCES

1. Daiger, S.P., Heckenlively, J.R, Lewis, R.A, and Pelias, M.Z., DNA linkage studies of degenerative retinal diseases, in Degenerative Retinal Disorders: Clinical and Laboratory Investigations, Hollyfield, J.G., and LaVail, M.W., Eds., Alan R. Liss, 1987, 147.
2. Daiger, S.P., Humphries, .M.M, Sharp, E., McWilliams, P., Farrar, J., Bradley, D., McConnel, D.C., Kenna, P., Sparkes, R.S., Spence, M.A., Heckenlively, J.R., and Humphries, P., Linkage analysis of human chromosome 4: exclusion of autosomal dominant retinitis pigmentosa (ADRP) and detection of new linkage groups, Cytogenet. Cell Genet., 50, 181, 1989.
3. Smith, R.J.H., Holcomb, J.D., Daiger, S.P., Caskey, C.T, Pelias, M.Z., Alford, B.R., Fontenot, D.D., and Hejtmancik, J.F., Exclusion of the Usher's syndrome gene from much of chromosome 4, Cytogenet. Cell Genet., 50, 102, 1989.
4. Spence, M.A., Sparkes, R.S., Heckenlively, J.R., Pearlman, Zedalis, D., Sparkes, M., Crist, M., and Tideman, S., Probable genetic linkage between autosomal dominant retinitis pigmentosa (RP) and amylase (Amy$_2$): evidence of an RP locus on chromosome 1, Amer. J. Hum. Genet., 29, 397, 1977.
5. Field, L.L., Heckenlively, J.R., Sparker, R.S., Garcia, C.A., Farson, C., Zedalis, D., Sparkes, M.C., Crist, M., Tidemsn, S., and Spence, M.A., Linkage analysis of five pedigrees affected with typical autosomal dominant retinitis pigmentosa, J. Med. Genet., 19, 266, 1982.
6. Heckenlively, J.R., Pearlman, J.T., Sparkes, R.S., Spence, M.A., Zedalis, D., Field, L., Sparkes, M.A., Crist, M., and Tideman, S., Possible assignment of a dominant retinitis pigmentosa gene to chromosome 1, Ophthalmic Res., 14, 46, 1982.
7. Klopfer, H.W., Laquaite, J.K., and McLaurin, J.W., The hereditary syndrome of congenital deafness and retinitis pigmentosa, Laryngoscope, 76, 850, 1966.
8. Pelias, M.Z., Lemoine, D.R, Kossar, A.L., Ward, L.J., Wilson, A.F., and Elston, R.C., Linkage studies of Usher's syndrome: analysis of an Acadian kindred in Louisiana, Cytogenet. Cell Genet., 47, 111, 1988.
9. Smith, R.J.H, Holcomb, J.D., Caskey, C.T., Pelias, M.Z., and Daiger, S.P, Multipoint linkage analysis of Usher syndrome: exclusion of chromosome 4, Amer. J. Hum. Genet., 43, A159, 1988.
10. Smith, R.J.H., Herrera, C.A., Pelias, M.Z., Kimberling, W.J, Daiger, S.P., and Hejtmancik, J.F., Multipoint analysis of Ushers syndrome: exclusion of chromosomes 6, 17 and 19, Amer. J. Hum. Genet., 45, A163, 1989.
11. Smith, R.J.H., Pelias, M.Z., Daiger, S.P., Herrera, C.H., Kimberling, W.J., and Hejtmancik, J.F., Clinical and genetic heterogeneity within the Acadian Usher population, submitted Amer. J. Hum. Genet., 1990.
12. Pelias, M.Z., Smith, R.J.H., Daiger, S.P., and Hejtmancik, J.F., Usher syndrome in Louisiana, in press, Proc. 6th World Congress of the International Retinitis Pigmentosa Association, 1990.
13. Daiger, S.P., Appendix H. The Retinitis Pigmentosa (RP) Collection, NIH Publication No. 89-2011, 1988/1989 Catalog of Cell Lines, NIGMS Human Genetic Mutant Cell Repository, 599, 1988.
14. NIH Publication No. 89-2011, 1988/1989 Catalog of Cell Lines, NIGMS Human Genetic Mutant Cell Repository, 1988.

15. Heckenlively, J.R., Rodriguez, J.A., and Daiger, S.P., Autosomal dominant sector retinitis pigmentosa: two families with rhodopsin codon 23 transversion, in press, Arch. Ophthal., 1990.

16. Myers, R.H., Leavitt, J., Farrer, L.A., Jagadeesh, J., McFarlan, H., Mastromauro, C.A., Mark, R.J., and Gusella, J.F., Homozygotes for Huntington disease, Amer. J. Hum. Genet., 45, 615, 1989.

17. Reed-Fourquet, L.L., and Daiger, S.P., Implementation of LIPED on a Cray X-MP Supercomputer, Amer. J. Hum. Genet., 45, A158, 1989.

18. Erratum, Amer. J. Hum. Genet., 29, 592, 1977.

19. Ott, J., Analysis of Human Genetic Linkage, Baltimore, Johns Hopkins University Press, 1985.

20. Lathrop, G.M., Lalouel, J.M., Julier, C., and Ott, J., Strategies for multilocus linkage analysis in humans, Proc. Natl Acad. Sci., 81, 3433, 1984.

21. Boehnke, M. and Ploughman, J., Estimating the power of a proposed linkage study: a practical computer simulation, Amer. J. Hum. Genet., 36, 513, 1986.

22. McWilliams, P., Farrar, G.J., Kenna, P., Bradley, D.G., Humphries, M.M, Sharp, E.M., McConnell, D.J., Lawler, M., Shields, D., Ryan, C., Stephens, K., Daiger, S.P., and Humphries, P., Autosomal dominant retinitis pigmentosa (ADRP): localization of an ADRP gene to the long arm of chromosome 3, Genomics, 5, 619, 1989.

23. Nakamura, Y., Leppert, M., O'Connell, P., Wolfe, R., Holm, T., Culver, M., Martin, C., Fujimoto, E., Hoff, M., Kumlin, E., and White, R., Variable number of tandem repeat (VNTR) markers for human gene mapping, Science, 235, 1616, 1987.

24. Saiki, R.K., Gelfand, D.H., Stoffel, S., Scharf, S.J., Higuchi, R., Horn, G.T., Mullis, K.B., and Erlich, H.A., Primer-directed enzymatic amplification of DNA with a thermostable DNA polymerase, Science, 239, 487, 1988.

25. Rodriguez, J.A.,and Daiger, S.P., Application of polymerase chain reaction (PCR) methodology to hypervariable loci in humans, Proc. Ann. Mtng, Texas Genetics Society, 16, 17, 1989.

26. Rodriguez, J.A., Blanton, S.H., and Daiger, S.P., The polymerase chain reaction and a candidate gene approach to mapping autosomal dominant retinitis pigmentosa, Proc. Ann. Mtng, Texas Genetics Society, 17, 10, 1990.

27. Laidlaw, J.L., Rodriguez, J.A., Cottingham, A.W., Blanton, S.H., Reed-Fourquet, L.L., and Daiger, S.P., Rapid linkage analysis of type II autosomal dominant retinitis pigmentosa (ADRP) using the polymerase chain reaction (PCR), in press, Amer. J. Hum. Genet., 1990.

28. Rodriguez, J.A., Liou, G.I., and Daiger, S.P., Enhanced detection of an RFLP at the interstitial retinol binding protein (RBP3) locus, in press, Nuc. Acids Res., 1990.

29. Daiger, S.P., Giesenschlag, N., Cottingham, A.W., Reed-Fourquet, L.L., Sparkes, R.S., Spence, M.A., and Heckenlively, J.R., Exclusion of autosomal dominant retinitis pigmentosa from linkage to the Rh blood group, Amer. J. Hum. Genet., 45, A136, 1989.

30. Bradley, D.G., Farrar, G.J., Sharp, E.M., Kenna, P., Humphries, M.M., McConnell, D.J., Daiger, S.P., McWilliams, P., and Humphries, P., Autosomal dominant retinitis pigmentosa: exclusion of the gene from the short arm of chromosome 1 including the region surrounding the rhesus locus, Amer. J. Hum. Genet., 44, 570, 1989.

31. Blanton, S.H., Cottingham, A.W., Giesenschlag, N., Heckenlively, J.R., Humphries, P., and Daiger, S.P., Further evidence of exclusion of linkage between type II autosomal dominant retinitis pigmentosa (ADRP) and D3S47 on 3q, in press, <u>Genomics</u>, 1990.

32. Blanton, S.H., Cottingham, A.W., Laidlaw, J.L., Heckenlively, J.R., and Daiger, S.P., Exclusion map of type II autosomal dominant retinitis pigmentosa (ADRP), in press, <u>Amer. J. Hum. Genet.</u>, 1990.

33. Edwards, J.H., Exclusion mapping, J. Med. Genet., 24, 539, 1987.

34. Dryja, T.P., McGee, T.L., Reichel, E., Hahn, L.B., Cowley, G.S., Yandell, D.W., Sandberg, M.A., and Berson, E.L., A point mutation on the rhodopsiin gene in one form of retinitis pigmentosa, <u>Nat</u>. 343, 364, 1990.

35. Rodriguez, J.A., Garcia, C.A., Lewis, R.A., Heckenlively, J.R., and Daiger, S.P., Screening a mutation in the first exon of the rhodopsin gene using allele specific oligonucleotide (ASO) hybridization, in press, <u>Amer. J. Hum. Genet.</u>, 1990.

36. Heckenlively, J.R., Autosomal dominant retinitis pigmentosa, in <u>Retinitis Pigmentosa</u>, Heckenlively, J.R., Ed., J.B. Lippincott, 1988, 146.

INDIAN PEDIGREES WITH RECESSIVE RETINITIS PIGMENTOSA: POTENTIAL FOR HOMOZYGOSITY MAPPING

[1]Chand, A., [2]Kumaramanickavel, G., [3]Abraham, M., [4]Gahlot, D. K., [5]Apte, B. N. and [1]Denton, M. J.

[1] Biochemistry Department, University of Otago, Dunedin , New Zealand.
[2] Institute of Physiology and Experimental Medicine , Madras Medical College, Madras, India.
[3] Medical Research Foundation, 18 College Road Madras, India.
[4]Taparia Institute of Ophthalmology, Bombay Hospital, Bombay, India.
[5] Medical Genetic Unit, Bombay Hospital, Bombay, India.

1. ABSTRACT

A high proportion of individuals with recessive retinitis pigmentosa (RP) in India are the children of consanguineous marriages. The most common type of consanguineous marriages are first cousin and uncle-niece. Such individuals provide the basis for a novel approach to mapping the genes responsible for recessive diseases know as 'homozygosity mapping'. Here we describe briefly the method of homozygosity mapping and present a number of consanguineous Indian recessive RP pedigrees which are currently being subjected to this type of gene mapping with a view to determining the number and location of the genes responsible for recessive RP.

2. INTRODUCTION

The 'standard' method of searching for genes responsible for genetic disease using RFLPs as linked markers, which has been successfully applied to locate the chromosomal position of the genes responsible for a number of diseases including Huntington's Disease[1], cystic fibrosis[2], and Duchenne muscular dystrophy[3], has generally depended on combining the linkage data from several families with the disease, each family having two or more affected individuals, a procedure which generally necessitates the collection of blood specimens from many individuals in each family.

Unfortunately this standard approach is often difficult to apply, particularly in the case of recessive diseases because it is often difficult to find sufficient families with two or more affected individuals and generally logistically impossible to collect blood specimens from all the informative individuals in the pedigree. A novel search strategy which can be used to map recessive genes which also uses RFLPs as linked markers but largely circumvents this problems is known as 'homozygosity mapping'. Here we describe this method briefly and discuss its potential application to mapping the recessive RP genes.

3. HOMOZYGOSITY MAPPING

In a child with a recessive disease whose parents are related, a region of several centimorgans on either side of the disease gene will nearly always be homozygous by descent[4]. Many other regions will also be homozygous by descent. For example, in the case of the child of a first cousin marriage as much as 1/16 of his entire genome will be homozygous by descent. Homozygosity mapping depends on the fact that the region containing a recessive gene will nearly always be homozygous by descent in unrelated inbred individuals with the disease, while other regions of homozygosity by descent will vary from individual to individual. Therefore any region of the genome which is tested for homozygosity in a number of unrelated inbred individuals with the disease and which appears to exhibit a higher frequency of homozygosity than that expected by chance is a putative site of the gene responsible for the recessive disease.

A very idealised illustration of the basic concept of homozygosity mapping is shown in Figure 1. The plot shows the hypothetical results which might be derived by homozygosity mapping of thirty unrelated individuals with recessive RP whose parents are first cousins. Each of the letters a, b, c etc represents the position of an RFLP within a hypothetical region of the genome X–Y. The RFLPs are assumed to be highly informative being homozygous in only 10% of the general population so that only 3 individuals will be expected to be homozygous for each RFLP by chance. In addition, 1/16 of the thirty individuals would also be expected to be homozygous by descent by chance for each RFLP, contributing further to the background level of homozygosity which in this hypothetical example is shown as ranging from 3 to 5 individuals. The two arrows indicate regions where the level of homozygosity is more than would be expected by chance, and such highly homozygous regions are possible locations of recessive RP genes.

Because this method of gene mapping only requires one blood specimen from one affected individual in each family, it is logistically far easier than the standard method. Moreover, as is indicated in Figure 1, the method will work even when there is heterozygosity if a large number of individuals are included in the study. Indeed, as the number of individuals included increases, it becomes possible not only to detect the position of more than one gene, but also to estimate the relative frequency of the various loci responsible for the disease by comparing the size of the peaks on the homozygous plot.

The fundamental problem with the method is that in the Western world where most of the clinical material for gene mapping purposes is drawn, the level of consanguinity is so low that the effort involved in collecting sufficient inbred cases with a particular recessive disease is prohibitive. However, there are regions where this is not a problem. In southern India for example, which has the highest percentage of inbred families in the world, mainly first cousin and uncle-niece marriages, [5,6] homozygosity mapping is a perfectly feasible strategy for locating the genes responsible for recessive diseases.

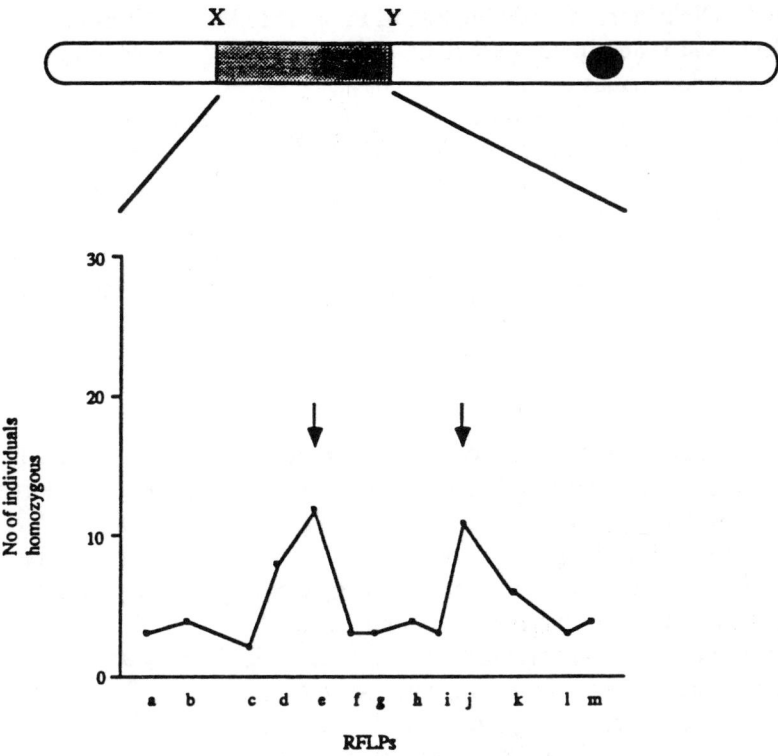

Figure 1   Homozygosity Plot

4. INDIAN RECESSIVE RETINITIS PIGMENTOSA

Because of the high incidence of consanguineous marriages in the general population in India, one would predict, on basic Mendelian grounds, that of the three genetic types of RP, autosomal dominant, autosomal recessive and X-linked recessive, the proportion of recessive RP, compared with the other types, would be far higher than in most Western countries.

This is certainly the impression gained by one of us (DKG) after nearly two decades of clinical experience in Delhi and Bombay. The same impression was also gained by two of use (AC and MJD) during a three month period from March to May 1990. while interviewing RP patients in Bombay made known to us by DKG and by the Indian RP society. None of the families ascertained in Bombay during this period could be definitely classified as either X-linked recessive, or autosomal dominant. Further evidence that the proportion of recessive RP in India, compared to other types of RP, is higher than in most other countries and that the high level of consanguinity is the likely cause, is provided by a study carried out by one of us (GK) on forty-seven consecutive unrelated cases of RP referred to the Government Ophthalmological Hospital in Madras over a two year period between 1986 and 1988. In this particular study, consanguinity was found to be present in 31 of the 47 families, an astonishingly high 69%.

Again, in none of these 47 families was the genetic type X-linked recessive, and in only two families, 4% was the genetic type found to be autosomal dominant. This very low percentage of only 4%, where the transmission was definitely 'non autosomal recessive' ie X-linked recessive or autosomal dominant, contrasts with the much higher levels generally seen in Europe and the USA[7,8]. Also, the level of consanguinity of 69% contrasts dramatically with the figure of only 6.8% found in a recent study in the UK[7].

5. CONCLUSION

The very high proportion of all Indian RP cases which are consanguineous autosomal recessive makes India, and particularly southern India, an ideal place to collect a large number of cases for homozygosity mapping of the recessive RP genes. Towards this end we have commenced working out the pedigrees of patients with RP in Bombay and Madras to find suitable individuals with recessive RP from consanguineous families. Some of the pedigrees already worked out are shown in Figure 2.

Pedigrees B1 and B2 are from the Parsi community in Bombay and illustrate the extremely complex patterns of consanguinity commonly seen in various ethnic and social groups in the subcontinent. Pedigrees B3 and B4 are Muslim families from Bombay. Pedigrees M1, 2, 3, 4 and 5 are Hindu families from Madras. Blood specimens have been collected from at least one affected inbred individual in all the families shown and several more consanguineous recessive RP families are currently being ascertained in Madras, Vellore and Ahmedabad. Hopefully this application of homozygosity mapping to locate the genes responsible for recessive RP will contribute substantially over the next few years to our understanding of the molecular genetics of the disease.

6. ACKNOWLEDGEMENTS

We wish to thank the British Retinitis Pigmentosa Society and the West Australian Retinitis Pigmentosa Foundation from providing the funds to support this project. We also wish to thank the President of the Vision Research Foundation and the Director of Scientific Studies of the Medical Research Foundation at the Sankara Nethralaya in Madras for their assistance and collaboration in the initiation of the project, and the Medical Director of the Bombay Hospital for his assistance in making available at the Bombay Hospital, facilities for DNA extraction.

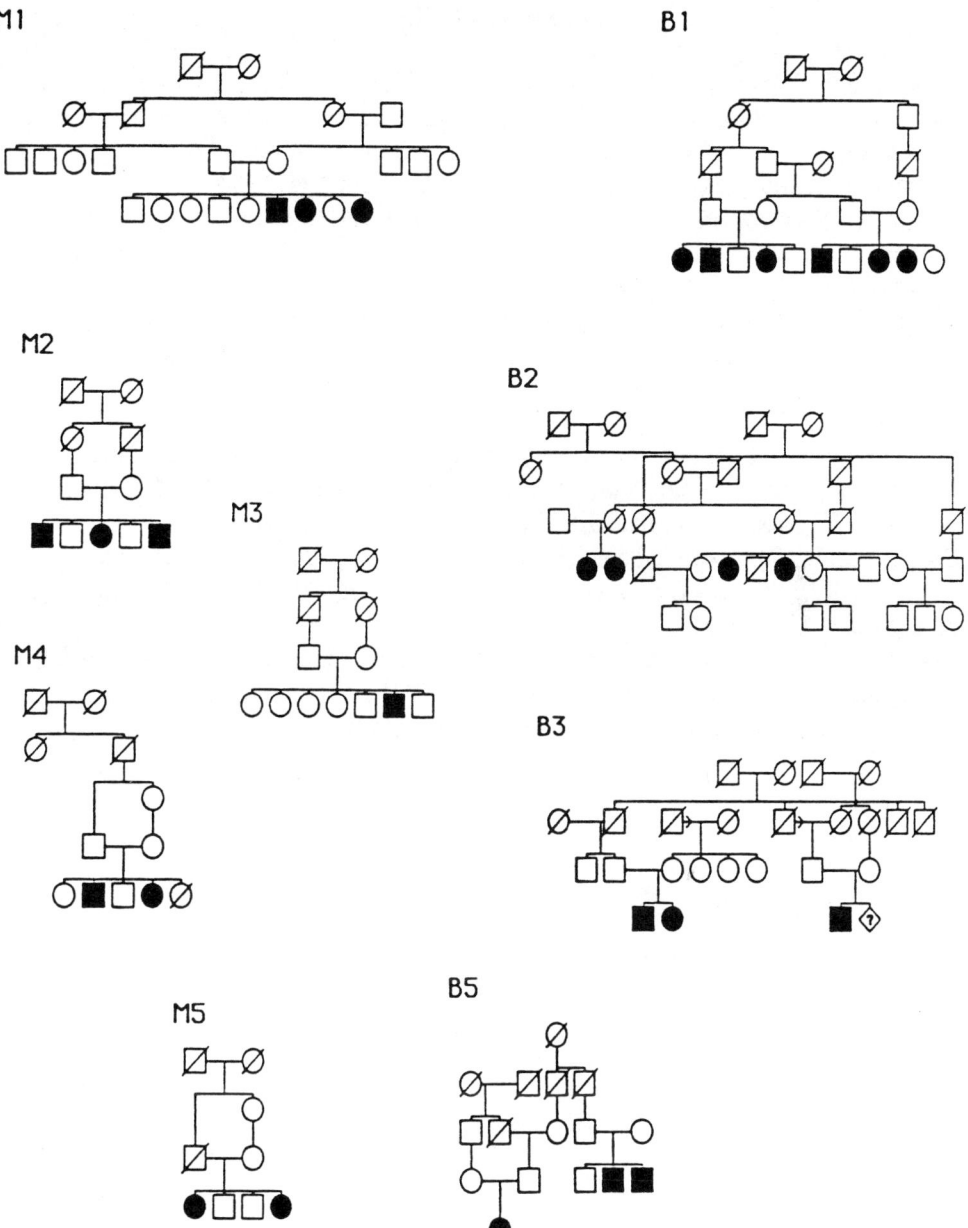

Figure 2 Consanguineous Indian Pedigrees with Recessive Retinitis Pigmentosa

7. REFERENCES

1   Gusella, J.F., Wexler, N. S., Conneally, P.M., Naylor, S. L., Anderson, M. A., Tanzi, R. E., Watkins, P. C., Ottina, K., Wallace, M.R., Sakaguchi, A Y., Young, A. B., Shoulson, I., Bonilla, E. and Martin, J. B., A polymorphic DNA marker genetically linked to Huntington's disease, *Nature* 306, 234, 1983.

2   White, R., Woodward, S., Leppert, M., O'Connell, P., Hoff, M., Herbst, J., Lalouel, J. M., Dean, M. and Vande Woude, C., A closely linked genetic marker for cystic fibrosis, *Nature* 318, 382, 1985.

3   Davies, K. E., Pearson, P.L., Harper, P. S., Murray, J. M., O'Brien, T., Sarfarzi, M.and Williamson, R., Linkage analysis of two cloned DNA sequences flanking the Duchene muscular dystrophy locus on the short arm of the human X chromosome, *Nucleic Acids Res* 11, 2303, 1983.

4   Lander, E. S. and Botstein, D., Homozygosity mapping : A way to map human recessive traits with the DNA of inbred children, *Science* 236,1567, 1987.

5   Sanghvi, L.D., Inbreeding in India, *Eug Quart*, 13, 291, 1966.

6   Sanghvi, L. D., The genetic consequences of inbreeding, *The Role of natural Selection in Human Evolution*, ed Salzano, F.M., North -Holland Publishing Co, Amsterdam, 1975, 323.

7   Jay, M On the heredity of retinitis pigmentosa, Br J. Ophthalmolgy, 6, 405, 1982.

8   Broughman, J.A., Coneally, P. M.and Nance, W. E., Population genetic studies of retinitis pigmentosa, *Am J. Hum Genet* 32, 223, 1980.

Autosomal dominant retinitis pigmentosa (RP4): Analysis of mutations within the Rhodopsin gene

GJ Farrar[1], P Kenna[1], R Redmond[2], P McWilliam[1],
DG Bradley[1], MM Humphries[1], EM Sharp[1],
Fishman G[3], Marchese C[4], Fusi L[4], Dufier JL[5],
Abitbol M[5] and Humphries P[1]

1. Department of Genetics, Trinity College Dublin, Dublin 2, Ireland.
2. Department of Medical Genetics, The Queen's University of Belfast, City Hospital, Lisburn Road, Belfast, Northern Ireland.
3. Department of Ophthalmology, Eye and Ear Hospital, 1855 West Taylor St., Chicago, Illinois 60612, USA.
4. Labortorio Analisi, Ospdale Mauriziano, Largo Turati 62, I 100100 Torino, Italy.
5. INSERM, Hospital Necker-Enfants-Malades, 149 rue de Sevres, 757143 Paris Cedex 15, France .

Summary

Base substitutions in exon 1 at codons 23 and 58, in exon 5 at codon 347 and a deletion in exon 4 at codons 255 / 256 of the rhodopsin gene have previously been observed in varying proportions of autosomal dominant retinitis pigmentosa (ADRP) patients. The regions around the sites of these mutations in the rhodopsin gene have been amplified in affected individuals from 38 ADRP pedigrees including 22 of Irish origin representing approximately 70% of the ADRP population in Ireland. These were analysed either by direct sequencing, allele specific oligonucleotide hybridisation (ASO), single strand conformation gel analysis (SSCPE) or restriction enzyme cutting in cases where the mutation either destroyed / created a restriction enzyme site. These mutations have been found to be absent in all Irish patients, including one pedigree in which the disease has been closely linked to the rhodopsin gene. However the codon 58 mutation was observed in one American ADRP patient.

Introduction

Retinitis Pigmentosa describes a group of inherited retinopathies which are both clinically and genetically heterogeneous. They can be broadly divided into X-linked (XLRP), autosomal dominant (ADRP) and autosomal recessive (ARRP). However further genetic heterogeneity exists within these categories. For example the presence of two loci on the X chromosome separated by approximately 20 cM has been firmly established using pooled linkage data[1]. In the case of ADRP, the disease genes segregating in a number of families map close to the DNA marker D3S47 on 3q[2], whereas in other families the disease genes are excluded from the same region of 3q, providing evidence of genetic heterogeneity within ADRP[3,4]. Furthermore weak evidence for a second ADRP gene on 3q approximately 10cM from the first ADRP linkage has been reported[5].

Moreover the presence of intra-allelic genetic heterogeneity in ADRP has been established. A number of different mutations within the rhodopsin gene have been defined. The first of these a C-->A transversion at codon 23 of the rhodopsin gene, resulting in a proline -->histidine substitution was observed in approximately 12% of American ADRP patients [6]. More recently two C-->T transitions involving different nucleotides at codon 347 and a C-->G transversion at codon 58 have been found representing 6% of the same American ADRP population[7]. Furthermore a three base pair deletion spanning codons 255 / 256 has been observed in a single English ADRP pedigree[8]. In view of these data we have analysed the regions around these rhodopsin mutations in patients from 38 ADRP pedigrees including 22 of Irish origin to investigate if these previously defined mutations are present[9]. Included in this group is the original ADRP family in which the disease gene was first mapped [2] and in which the disease gene has since been shown to be significantly linked to rhodopsin at 0.00 recombination[3].

Materials and Methods

ADRP pedigrees:

22 pedigrees assessed for the rhodopsin mutations were of Irish origin and showed a probable autosomal dominant mode inheritance. The remaining 16 ADRP pedigrees were either of American, French or Italian origin.

The Irish ADRP pedigrees used in the analyses have been ascertained either through the Royal Victoria Eye and Ear Hospital, Dublin or the Royal Victoria Hospital, Belfast. Affected members exhibited classical changes characteristic of RP including night blindness, reduced peripheral visual fields, intraretinal bone-corpuscle pigmentary deposits in 360° of the retinal mid-periphery, waxy disc pallor, retinal vessel attenuation and reduced or extinguished ERGs. Together these two groups of ADRP patients are estimated to represent 70% of the population of ADRP patients in Ireland (Dr GJ Farrar, Dr B Page, Dr R Redmond, unpublished).

PCR amplification:

PCR amplifications were performed in reactions containing 0.5-1.0ug of genomic DNA, 50mM KCL, 10 mM Tris-HCL pH 8.3 and 1.0-5.0 mM $MgCl_2$. Primers at positions 192-111 and 391-410, 301-320 and 681-700, 4125-4144 and 4241-4260 and 5145-5164 and 5279-5298 were designed to amplify the region around codon 23, codon 58, codons 255/256 and codon 347 respectively[10].

Methods for analyses of rhodopsin mutations:

Direct sequencing:

PCR amplified DNA was chloroform extracted, treated with Proteinase K, phenol / chloroform extracted, chloroform extracted, spun through a Sepharose CL-6B column and then ethanol precipitated[11]. The region around the codon 23 mutation was sequenced using a nested primer (at position 301-320) within the amplified fragment. 1-2 pmol (p-32) of end-labelled sequencing primer was combined with 250-500ng of the amplified, purified DNA template and heat denatured at $94^{\circ}C$ for 5 mins. The T7 DNA Polymerase Sequencing System (Promega) was then followed with the omission of the labelling step. Samples were heat denatured at $70^{\circ}C$ for 5 mins prior to running on 6% polyacrylamide sequencing gels and then autoradiographed for 1-2 days at $-70^{\circ}C$.

Restriction enzyme digestion:

The codon 58 mutation created a Dde I restriction site. Similarly both codon 347 mutations destroy the recognition sequence for the restriction endonuclease Msp I. Hence these mutations were assessed directly by PCR amplification of the region around these mutations, followed by cutting with the appropriate restriction enzyme and running on 2% agarose gels. A 154bp fragment around codon 347 was amplified and cut with MspI, the normal and mutant sequences produce fragments of 27bp x2 and 100bp or 27bp and 127bp respectively. Similarly a 400bp fragment around codon 58 was amplified and cut with Dde I, the normal and mutant sequences produce fragments of 310bp and 90 bp or 235bp, 90bp and 75bp respectively.

Allele Specific Oligonucleotide Hybridisation (ASO):

Amplified products were DOT blotted onto Hybond-N, and hybridised to both mutant and wild type ASO. The ASOs for codon 23 was made at position 354-373 the mutant containing the C-->A transversion at position 362 and the ASOs for the 255/256 deletion were at position 4154-4173 (wild type) and position 4153-4175 (mutant), the mutant missing 3 bases at position 4166-4168. Filters for the codon 23 mutation were washed in 2x SSC at room temp for 10', 2x SSC at 55°C for 20' and then 2x SSC at 62°C for 10'. Filters for the codons 255/256 deletion were washed in 2x SSC at room temp for 10' and then 2x SSC at 60°C for 10'.

Single Strand Conformational Analyses (SSCP):

PCR amplifications were performed using 10pmol of end labelled primer (as above). 1ul of the amplified product was mixed with 100ul of 0.1% SDS and 10mM EDTA. 2ul of the resulting solution was mixed with 2ul of 95% formamide, 20mMEDTA, 0.05% bromophenol blue and 0.05% xylene cyanol, heated denatured at 80°C for 5' and run on a 6% polyacrylamide gel containing 10% glycerol at 4°C[12].

Results and Discussion

The regions around the previously defined rhodopsin mutations at codon 23, 58, 255/256 and 347 have been analysed in ADRP patients. The codon 23 mutation was analysed either by direct sequencing, single strand conformation analyses or allele specific oligonucleotide hybridisation, the codon 58 and 347 mutations by restriction enzyme digestion and the codon 255/256 deletion by allele specific oligonucleotide hybridisation. 38 ADRP pedigrees have been screened for these mutations, 22 of which are of Irish origin and represent approximately 70% of the ADRP population in Ireland. To date in our analyses none of these known mutations have been found in our 22 Irish pedigrees. However we have found one family of American origin with the codon 58 mutation (Fig: 1).

Interestingly the codon 23 mutation previously observed in 12% of an American population of ADRP patients, many of whom were of British ancestry[6], has not been found in this Irish ADRP population. Moreover this mutation is not present in a total of 98 ADRP families of European origin[9]. Hence if the rhodopsin codon 23 mutation is present in the European ADRP population it is extremely rare. The variation in the frequency of the codon 23 mutation between the American and European populations would lead one to speculate that the higher frequency found in the American population may be the result of a founder effect. Such effects have been observed for example in the Porphyria Variegata population in South Africa[13] and the Huntington Chorea population in Venezuala[14]. This is supported by recent data indicating that the 17 ADRP patients found to contain the codon 23 mutation in the original American study show linkage disequilibrium with two neutral polymorphisms in the rhodopsin gene, indicating that these patients

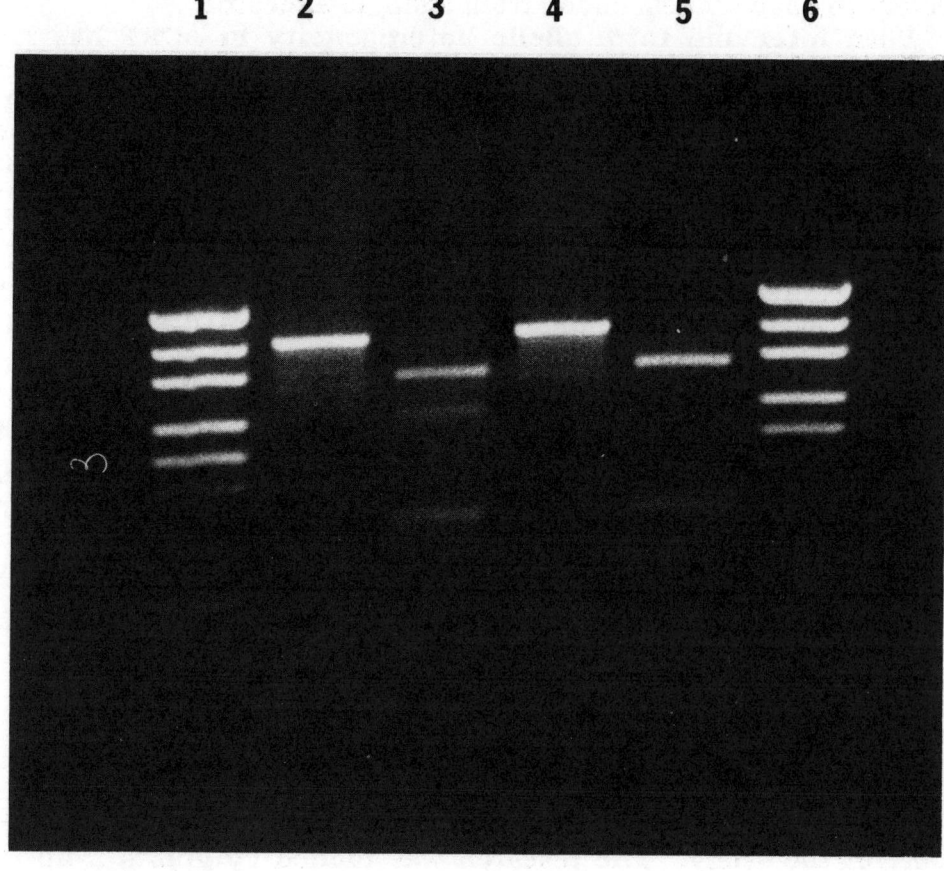

Figure 1:

Lanes 1and 6 contain Msp I cut PUC 19, lanes 2 and 4 contain uncut DNA from two ADRP patients, lanes 3 and 5 contain DNA cut with Dde I from the same two patients. The patient in lane 5 has the normal sequence around codon 58, resulting in fragments of 310bp and 90bp, whereas the patient in lane 3 has the codon 58 mutation resulting in the creation of a Dde I site and the presence of additional fragments of 235bp and 75bp. Note the 90bp and 75bp fragments are difficult to visualise in this photograph.

are likely to have all descended from a single ancestor[7].

Both inter and intra allelic heterogeneity in ADRP has now been firmly established. Mutations in the rhodopsin gene have been found to account for approximately 18% of ADRP cases in one American ADRP population, however to date in European populations detected rhodopsin mutations account for very few of the ARDP cases observed. Extensive analyses of these patients will be required to investigate the possibility of as yet unidentified mutations in rhodopsin and to identify mutations in other genes which also result in ADRP. There are many previously identified genes which could be considered as possible candidate genes for both ADRP and ARRP. Examples are the rod specific alpha subunit of transducin[15] which also maps to chromosome 3, the beta subunit of c-GMP phosodiesterase which has been implicated as the causative gene in the rd mouse[16] and many of the other participants in the visual excitation pathway. Future analyses of these genes in large populations of RP patients must inevitably lead us to a greater understanding of the underlying pathogenesis of this heterogeneous group of retinopathies.

Acknowledgments

Many thanks once again to the RP families for their continuing support in the study. The research was funded by grants from the National RP Foundation of America, RP Ireland-Fighting Blindness, the British Retinitis Pigmentosa Society, the George Gund Fund, and Wellcome Trust.

References

1. Ott J, Bhattacharya S, Chen JD, Denton MJ, Donald J, Duba C, Farrar GJ, et al. Localization of multiple retinitis pigmentosa loci on the X chromosome. Proc Natl Acad Sci 87: 701-704, 1990.

2. McWilliam P, Farrar GJ, Kenna P, Bradley DG, Humphries MM, Sharp EM, McConnell DJ, et al. Autosomal dominant retinitis pigmentosa (ARDP): Localization of an ADRP gene to the long arm of chromosome 3. Genomics 5: 619-622, 1989.

3. Farrar G J, McWilliam P, Bradley D G, Kenna P, Lawler M, Sharp E M, Humphries M M, Eiberg H, Conneally P M, Trofatter J A and Humphries P. Autosomal dominant retinitis pigmentosa: Linkage to Rhodopsin and evidence for genetic heterogeneity. Genomics 1990

4. Inglehearn CF, Jay M, Lester DH, Bashir R, Jay B, Bird AC, Wright AF, et al. No evidence for linkage between late onset autosomal dominant retinitis pigmentosa and chromosome 3 locus D3S47 (C17): Evidence for genetic heterogeneity. Genomics 6: 168-173, 1990.

5. Olsson JE, Samanna CH, Jimenez J, Pongratz J, Chand A, Watty A, Seuchter SA, et al. Gene of Type II autosomal dominant retinitis pigmentosa maps on the long arm of chromosome 3. Amer J Med Genet 1990.

6. Dryja TD, McGee TL, Reichel E, Hohn LB, Cowley GS, Yandell DN, Sandberg MA, et al. A point mutation of the rhodopsin gene in one form of retinitis pigmentosa. Nature 343: 364-366, 1990.

7. Dryja TP, McGee TL, Hahn LB, Cowley GS, Olsson JE, Reichel E, Sandberg MA, and Berson EL. Mutations within the rhodopsin gene in patients with autosomal dominant retinitis pigmentosa. New Eng J Med., 323 (19), 1990.

8. Inglehern CF, Bashir R, Leister DH, Jay M, Bird AC and Bhattacharya S. A 3bp deletion in the rhodopsin gene in a family with autosomal dominant retinitis pigmentosa. Am J Hum Genet 48: 26-30 1991

9. Farrar GJ, Kenna P, Redmond R, McWilliam P, Bradley D, Humphries MM, Sharp EM, Inglehern CF, Bashir R, Jay M, Watty A, Ludwig M, Schinzel A, Samanns C, Gal A, Bhattacharya S, and Humphries P. Autosomal Dominant Retinitis Pigmentosa: Absence of the Rhodopsin Proline-->Histidine substitution (codon 23) in pedigrees from Europe. Am J Hum Genet 47 941-945 1990.

10. Nathans J and Hogness D S. Isolation and nucleotide sequence of the gene encoding human rhodopsin. Proc Natl Acad Sci 81: 4851-4855, 1984.

11. Yandell, D.W., and Dryja, T.P. Detection of DNA sequence polymorphism by enzymatic amplification and direct genomic sequencing. Amer J Hum Genet 45: 547-555, 1989.

12. Orita V, Suzuki Y, Sekiya and Hayashi K. Rapid and sensitive detection of point mutations and DNA polymorphisms using the polymerase chain reaction. Genomics 5 874-879 1989.

13. Dean G. (1971). Porphyria Varigata. In: 'The Porphyrias, a story of inheritance and environment', 2ed. Pitman Press, London, pp 4-13

14. Gusella JF, Wexler NS, Conneally PM, Naylor SL, Anderson MA, Tanzi RE. Watkins PC, et al. A polymorphic DNA marker genetically linked to Huntington disease. Nature 306: 234-238, 1983.

15. Blatt C, Eversole-Cire P, Cohn H, Zollman S, Fournier REK, Mohandas LT, Nesbitt M, et al. Chromosomal localization of genes encoding guaine nucleotide-binding protein sub-units in mouse and human. Proc Nat Acad Sci USA 85: 7642-7646 1988.

16. Bowes C, Li T, Danciger M, Baxter LC, Applebury ML, and Farber D. Retinal degeneration in the rd mouse is caused by a defect in the beta subunit of rod cGMP-phosphodiesterase. Nature 347 677-680 1990.

LINKAGE ANALYSIS OF AUTOSOMAL DOMINANT CONGENITAL STATIONARY NIGHT BLINDNESS IN A LARGE CHINESE PEDIGREE

Fei Yijian, Luo Chengren, Li Anren, Zhou Jiumu, Huang Yongzhi,
Department of Ophthalmology, The First University Hospital, West China University of Medical Sciences, Chengdu, China.

I. INTRODUCTION

Congenital stationary night blindness (CSNB) is a group of inherited retinal disorders characterized by non progressive night blindness present after birth, normal light-vision, normal-appearing fundus and specific manifestations in electroretinographic and psychophysical testings. There are three modes of inheritance, that is, autosomal dominant, autosomal recessive, and X-linked recessive. The incidence of CSNB in China could be as high as 3.7 in 10,000 of the population. The autosomal dominant type of CSNB is the most common, with a prevalence of approximately 1/10,000. Since the famous French Nougaret family, affected with autosomal dominant CSNB, was first described by Cunier in 1838, [1-3] it has been taken as an excellent paradigm of autosomal dominant inheritance in human genetics. It is only in the last 35 years, however, that we have gained an understanding of the pathogenesis of the disease based on a series of electrophysiological and psychophysical studies on CSNB [4-7]. Recent progress in human gene mapping, especially the application of recombinant DNA techniques, has made more effective the establishment of genetic linkages between hereditary diseases and genetic markers and thereby the assignment of loci for such diseases to specific chromosomes. More recently, tight genetic linkage between the X-linked form of CSNB and an Xp11.3 DNA marker, DXS7, was found by Musarella and colleagues.[8] However, there are no reports to date of linkage studies of autosomal dominant forms of CSNB. In an attempt to map the gene responsible for autosomal dominant CSNB, linkage analysis was carried out with six autosomal markers in a large Chinese family affected with typical autosomal dominant CSNB.

II. MATERIALS AND METHODS

Family Studies

The Chinese CSNB pedigree (under study) encompasses seven generations known to be affected with autosomal dominant CSNB, with at least 57 affected members of which 47 are living. Most family members live in rural areas within about 50 km. of Chengdu. The proband of the pedigree came to the Genetic Clinic of our Department because of night blindness since birth and many members in his kindred have the same symptoms. After a thorough eye examination, the proband was confirmed to have been affected with congenital stationary night blindness, and subsequently, we started an investigation on this family. A comprehensive ophthalmologic examination was performed on members of this family, including visual acuity, color vision, anterior segments of the eyes, funduscopic evaluation, visual fields, dark adaptations and full-field electroretinograms. The general clinical features of patients in the Chinese CSNB family consistently include congenital nonprogressive night blindness, without any disturbances in visual acuity, color vision and visual field. The fundi are normal of appearance, but loss of rod functions was well demonstrated in testings of adaptations and full-field ERGs. Specific clinical details will be presented elsewhere (Fei, et al. in preparation).

Typing of Genetic Markers

For the purpose of this study, blood samples were acquired from 37 family members in which 20 are affected. Patient's red cells were tested for blood groups including the ABO, the MN, the P and the Rhesus (Rh) system using the standard red blood cell typing techniques of our Genetic Laboratory. The designation Rh positive or negative is derived from whether the Rh D type tests positive or negative to the anti-D serum. Phosphoglucomutase-1 (PGM1) and phosphogluconate dehydrogenase of red cells were determined in our laboratory using the method of horizontal starch-gel electrophoresis, which was first described by Spencer (1964).[9]

Linkage Analysis

Linkage analysis was performed on an IBM/PC Computer. Two-point recombination fractions were calculated using a LODS program.[10] Individual Rh antigen types as well as combinations of antigen types of Rh factor were analyzed for linkage.

III Results

Results of pairwise linkage analysis between autosomal dominant CSNB and 6 autosomal markers are listed in table 1.

Table 1, Lod Scores between Autosomal Dominant CSNB and Genetic Markers

Marker	Chromosome	θ (θm=θf)						Maximums	
		.00	.05	.10	.20	.30	.40	Z	θ
Rh (all types)	1	- ∞	- 0.09	- 0.05	0.40	0.33	0.05	0.41	0.22
RhC	1	- ∞	- 0.39	0.01	0.20	0.15	0.05	0.20	0.21
RhE	1	- ∞	- 0.51	- 0.06	0.20	0.18	0.01	0.22	0.24
PGM1	1	- ∞	- 2.6	- 1.6	- 0.64	- 0.09	- 0.05	- 0.01	0.48
PGD	1	- ∞	- 0.09	0.07	0.40	0.34	0.13	0.41	0.22
ABO	9	- ∞	- 4.08	- 2.48	-1.06	- 0.41	- 0.10	- 0.01	0.48
P	6	- ∞	0.96	1.15	0.96	0.26	0.17	1.15	0.11
MN	4	- ∞	- 3.6	- 2.2	-0.97	- 0.38	- 0.09	- 0.01	0.48

For simplicity, we report lod scores calculated at recombination fraction θ male = θ female. No statistically significant lod score was produced. The largest score is 1.1497 for CSNB-P at θ =0.1075. This level of score is a weak suggestion that a linkage may exist between autosomal dominant CSNB and the P locus. Both of the overall Rh group and PGD show positive maximal scores of 0.41 at θ =0.22, which do not reach the standard levels for establishing or rejecting linkage. Linkage could be excluded at values of θ=0.10 or less for CSNB and ABO, as well as MN. Close linkage between CSNB and PGM1 could also be excluded in this family.

IV. Discussion

The first description of congenital stationary night blindness can be traced back to 1838, when Cunier reported the Nougaret family dating to the 17th century, affected with autosomal dominant CSNB. The Nougaret family encompasses over ten generations, and includes over 2000 members, of whom 139 were affected. This pedigree is one of the largest on record of dominant inheritance. [1] It has been known since the beginning of this century that CSNB can be inherited both as an autosomal recessive and sex-linked disease. The large Chinese CSNB pedigree covers seven generations and contains 57 patients, in which male-to-male transmission of CSNB was demonstrated and there are no known "skipped generations". Therefore, it is clear that the disorder in this family is the result of an autosomal dominant CSNB gene with nearly complete penetrance. A new classification for CSNB was proposed by Miyake and associates in 1986.[11] It includes a complete type which lacks rod function by ERG and adaptometry and an incomplete type which shows some rod functions. Differences in clinical manifestations between the two types suggest a different pathogenesis. However Khouri et al [2] found both types in the same X-linked CSNB family, which makes it unlikely that the two types are different clinical entities. In our CSNB family, both complete and incomplete types are also present, so it is obvious that the new classification does not signify genetic specificity. Noble and associates (1990) [3] reported three patients in a family affected with autosomal dominant CSNB who showed electronegative ERG which resembled the Schubert-Bornschein type, which has been previously reported to be seen only in X-linked and autosomal recessive CSNB. Therefore, it is evident that these different manifestations in ERG and dark adaptation do not represent different genetic entities. This disease, regardless of the type of inheritance, appears to be characterized by a severe rod-system abnormality in all patients with a frequent variable mild to moderate cone system abnormality in most. [1] The findings of normal concentration of rhodopsin and its normal regenerating rate by fundus Reflectometry in two patients argue against a photochemical basis for this disease. The one histological study to date rules out an obvious structural abnormality of any portion of the retina. Although defects of neurotransmission between the photoreceptor and bipolar cells was proposed, the genetic defect and the biochemical basis of this disease remain to be localized and defined.

Linkage analysis is a valuable means of mapping genes for inherited traits to specific chromosomes. Linkage studies on CSNB can help to more accurately classify this disease. Localizing the CSNB gene to a specific chromosome has the potential for detection of gene carriers, which would provide information that may be helpful for antenatal diagnosis. Ultimately, by knowing the location of the CSNB gene defect, it will be possible to identify the biochemical and/or structural expression of the defect, and the pathogenesis of this genetic retinal disease would be well illuminated.

To map the gene responsible for autosomal dominant CSNB, a genetic linkage study was performed on a large Chinese family with typical dominant CSNB. The results have shown that close linkage between autosomal dominant CSNB and markers of PGM1, ABO and MN could be excluded. Lod scores between this type of CSNB and markers of Rh and PGD on chromosome 1 are positive, but of no statistical significance. Further linkage studies, particularly involving the use of DNA markers, will be required in order to accurately localize the gene segregating in this large Chinese pedigree.

This study is supported by the Natural Science Foundation of China.

References:

1.   Krill A.E.: Congenital Stationary Night Blindness in "Hereditary Retinal and Choroidal Disease. VII: Clinical Characteristics". New York, Harper & Row, 1977, p.391-417.

2. Khouri G. et al: X-Linked Congenital Stationary Night Blindness: Review and report of a family with hyperopia. Arch. Ophthalmol. 106:1417, 1988.

3.   Noble, K.G. et al: Autosomal Dominant Congenital Stationary Night Blindness and Normal Fundus with an Electronegative electroretinogram. Am.J. Ophthalmol. 109: 44, 1990.

4. Carr, R.E. and Siegel, I.M.: Electrophysiologic aspects of several retinal diseases. Am.J. Ophthalmol. 58; 95, 1964.

5. Carroll, F.D. and Haig, C.: Congenital Stationary Night Blindness without ophthalmoscopic or other abnormalities. Trans.Am.Ophthalmol. Soc. 50: 193, 1952.

6. Riggs,L.A.: Electroretinography in cases of night blindness. Part II Am.J. Ophthalmol. 38:70, 1954.

7. Francois, J. et al: A new pedigree of idiopathic Congenital Night Blindness. Am.J. Ophthalmol. 59; 621, 1965.

8.   Musarella, M.A. et al: Assignment of the gene for X-linked Congenital Stationary Night Blindness (CSNB1) to human chromosome Xp11.3. Cytogenet and Cell genet. 51:1049, 1989.

9. Spencer, N. et al: Phosphoglucomutase polymorphism in man. Nature 204: 742, 1964.

10. Liu Xinhua, et al: A program for linkage analysis (LODs).   Acta Genetica Sinica 12:232, 1985.

11. Miyake, Y. et al: Congenital Stationary Night Blindness with negative electroretinogram Arch. Ophthalmol. 104: 1013, 1986.

12. Weleber, R.G., et al: Aland Island Eye Disease (Forsius Eriksson Syndrome) Associated with Contiguous Deletion Syndrome at X21: Similarity to Incomplete Congenital Stationary Night Blindness: Arch. Ophthamol. 21.

A GENE FOR AUTOSOMAL DOMINANT RETINITIS PIGMENTOSA IS CLOSELY LINKED TO D3S20 ON 3q

Ch. Samanns[1,2], A. Watty[1], A. Chand[3], J. Pongratz[1,2],
V. Colantuoni[4], M.J. Denton[5] and A. Gal[1,2]

Institute für Humangenetik der Universität, [1]Bonn and
[2]Lübeck, FRG, [3]Department of Pathology, Prince of Wales
Hospital, Sydney, Australia, [4]Dipartimento di Biochimica
e Biotecnologie Mediche, Universita di Napoli, Napoli,
Italy, [5]Department of Biochemistry, University of Otago,
Dunedin, New Zealand

SUMMARY

Recently it has been found that in the USA in about
12% of patients with autosomal dominant retinitis pigmentosa (ADRP) there is a point mutation in codon 23 of the
rhodopsin gene, which maps to 3q21-q24. Prior to this it
was reported that in a large Irish pedigree, in which a
severe form of ADRP was segregating (so called type I,
early onset, diffuse) the ADRP locus shows tight linkage
and no recombination to D3S47, a marker locus on chromosome 3, which is known to be closely linked to the rhodopsin locus.

We performed linkage analysis on two large
Australian families with ADRP. Previous studies of these
two families failed to detect the codon 23-mutation, and
although linkage between the disease locus and D3S47 was
demonstrated, it appeared to be less tight ($\Theta_{max}=0,08$)
than in the Irish pedigree. Here we report that close
linkage and no recombination ($\Theta_{max}=0,00/z=7,571$) have
been detected between the ADRP locus and D3S20 (CRI-
L1169) in both families. Also the locus for cellular retinol binding protein I (RBP1), mapped on 3q21-q22, shows
tight linkage and no recombination ($\Theta_{max}=0,00/z_{max}=4,086$)
with the ADRP locus in one of the families. In the second
family, however, close linkage between the ADRP locus and
RBP1 can be excluded ($z=-4,009$ at $\Theta=0,001$).

INTRODUCTION

Retinitis pigmentosa (RP) is a group of hereditary
degenerative diseases of the retina. RP is both genetically and clinically heterogeneous (for review see reference 1). As to the pattern of inheritance, autosomal dominant and recessive, and X-linked forms are known, but
further genetic heterogeneity within each of the traits
is also very likely. Determining the map position of the
disease locus/loci would aid resolution of genetic heterogeneity and, at the same time, is the first step toward
cloning the gene(s) and exploring the molecular defect(s)

causing the disease.

Recently it has been found that in the USA in about 12% of patients with autosomal dominant retinitis pigmentosa (ADRP) there is a point mutation in codon 23 of the rhodopsin gene,[2] which maps to 3q21-q24,[3] leading to a replacement of an amino acid in an evolutionary highly conserved region of the rhodopsin molecule. Prior to this it was reported that the ADRP locus is tightly linked to D3S47,[4] a marker locus on chromosome 3, in a large Irish pedigree, in which a severe form (so called type I, early onset, diffuse) ADRP was segregating. The D3S47 and rhodopsin loci have also been reported being closely linked.[5]

Here we report the results of linkage analysis with two DNA probes from 3q in 2 large Australian families with a milder form of ADRP. Also in these families, previous studies have indicated linkage between the disease locus and D3S47, although it appeared to be less tight ($\Theta_{max}=0,08$)[6,7] than in the Irish pedigree.

MATERIALS AND METHODS

Families

The two pedigrees studied here are illustrated in Figures 1 and 2. Pedigree 20 (Figure 1) has already been described extensively.[6,8] Although the majority of patients complained of night blindness from their second decade onwards, visual acuity was well preserved until late in life. The ADRP segregating in this family can be categorized as type II according to the currently used subdivisions.[9,10]

In family S. (Figure 2), there are 15 known affected members in four generations, corresponding to an approximately 50% incidence of the disease.

Detailed clinical information is available on seven patients, who show common features. Night blindness was present from a very early age, and on this basis, the diagnosis was often made in childhood or early teens. The loss of visual field became apparent in childhood or teens, and was a serious handicap by the late 20's. Often an infero-nasal island of peripheral field was retained. Visual acuity was variable, but could be well preserved beyond the age of 40.

Ophthalmic examination revealed a remarkably low prevalence of cataract: insignificant lens opacities were found in only one subject (at 45 years of age). Ophthalmoscopically, the characteristic waxy pallor of the optic discs was present, with peripapillary atrophy, particularly inferiorly, in adult patients. Maculopathy was visible in all patients in the form of a more or less pronounced bull's eye maculopathy. The retinal vessels were attenuated and, by adult life, became obliterated beyond the equator. An aquatorial band of chorioretinal atrophy with pigment clumping was present in all increasing in width with age. The electroretinogram (ERG) was extinguished by about 30 years in some of the patients, in others, the scotopic ERG was greatly but the photopic ERG only slightly reduced.

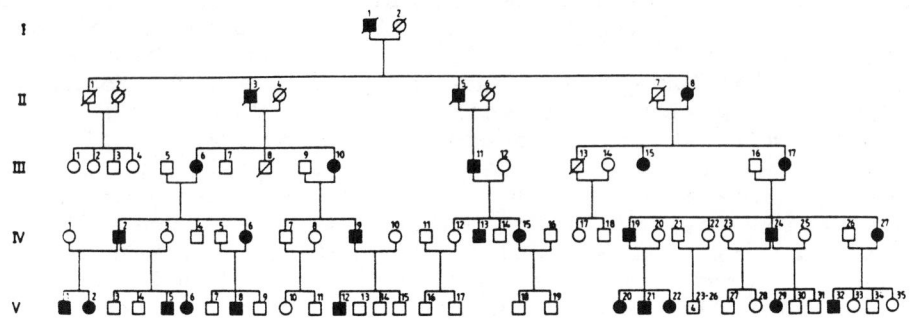

Figure 1. Pedigree 20

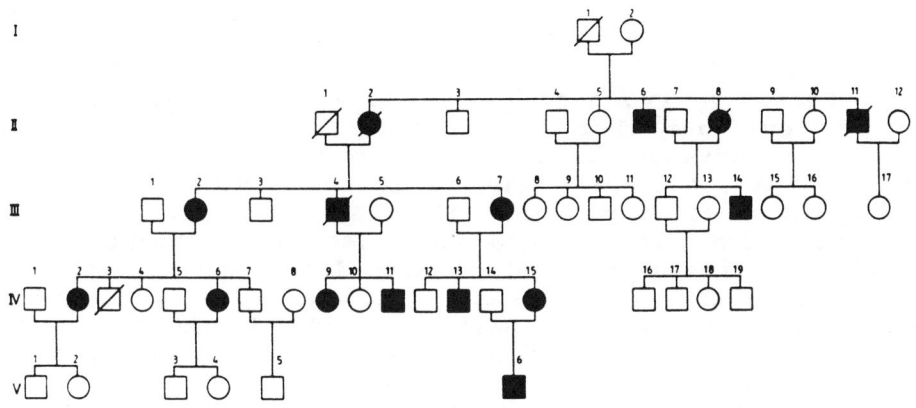

Figure 2. Family S

DNA studies

The methods for the extraction of DNA from whole blood, digestion of DNA with restrictrion enzymes, transfer onto nylon membranes, and Southern blot hybridization have been described previously.[11,12]

Probe CRI-L1169 was provided by Collaborative Research, Inc., Bedford (USA). The corresponding DNA locus (D3S20) has been mapped on chromosome 3.[3] After either MspI or BamHI digestion of genomic DNA, the probe detects allelic fragments and several invariable ones. In the present study, we used the BamHI RFLP with alleles C1 (about 12 kb) and C2 (about 11 kb).

The cDNA probe for the human cellular retinol binding protein I (CRBP) used is about 0,7 kb and contains the entire coding region bounded by 5'- and 3'-end untranslated sequences.[13] The corresponding locus (RBP1) has been mapped on 3q21-q22.[14] The probe detects a two-allele TaqI RFLP (A1/A2, 3,0 and 2,7 kb, respectively).[15]

The 1988 version of LIPED was used to compute the linkage data.[15] For our analysis, a mutation rate of 0,0003 and complete penetrance of the disease were assumed.

RESULTS

Results of pairwise linkage analyses are shown in Table 1. Since genetic heterogeneity in ADRP can not be excluded, the data obtained in the two families are presented separately. In both families, close linkage and no recombination have been found between the ADRP locus and D3S20 with maximum lod scores (z) of 5.825 and 1.746, respectively, at the recombination frequency (Θ) of 0,00. In pedigree 20, the locus (RBP1) for cellular retinol binding protein I also showed close linkage and no recombination (z_{max}=4,086 at Θ=0,00) to the disease locus, while in family S. several recombinations occured between these two loci and close linkage was excluded (z=-4,009 at Θ=0,001). Two-point linkage data further suggest that RBP1 and D3S20 must also be closely linked, since no recombination has been observed between them in 23 phase-known meioses (z_{max}=6,976 at Θ=0,00).

DISCUSSION

Recently, two different studies have provided independent evidence that a gene for ADRP maps on the long arm of chromosome 3. Firstly, it has been shown that there is a single-base change in the first exon of the rhodopsin gene,[2] mapped on 3q21-q24,[3] in about 12% of the patients with ADRP in the USA. Secondly, two-point and multipoint linkage data of a large Irish and British kindred showed that the disease locus was closely linked to both the D3S47 and rhodopsin loci.[5,17] Furthermore, neither of these two families have the codon 23-mutation found in the USA.[5] These data suggest that even if the disease in the British and Irish families was caused by a mutation in the rhodopsin gene, ADRP is genetically heterogeneous.

In the two Australian families studied here, it seems to be unlikely that ADRP is the consequence of a mutation in the rhodopsin gene. Firstly, no mutation in codon 23 was found in either of the families.[7] Secondly, close linkage to D3S47 (and, thus, also to rhodopsin) has been excluded. Accordingly, the data presented here strongly suggest that there are (at least) two genes in 3q, whose mutation leads to ADRP, i.e. in addition to probable allelic genetic heterogeneity of ADRP also a non-allelic one seems to be very likely. The question whether or not the disease gene is identical in the Irish, British, and 2 Australian families, can not be answered yet. Further studies in these and additional families are necessary to gain more information about the location of the gene or genes for ADRP on 3q and to confirm genetic heterogeneity.

TABLE 1

Results of Pairwise Linkage Analysis Between the ADRP, D3S20, and RBP1 Loci in 2 Australian Pedigrees With Autosomal Dominant Retinitis Pigmentosa[a]

ADRP vs D3S20

Θ_{max}	Z_{max}	z(0,00)	z(0,001)	z(0,05)	z(0,10)	z(0,20)	z(0,30)	z(0,40)
0,00	5,825	5,825	5,815	5,346	4,843	3,762	2,571	1,277[b]
0,00	1,746	1,746	1,743	1,624	1,613	1,282	0,966	0,525[c]

ADRP vs RBP1

Θ_{max}	Z_{max}	z(0,00)	z(0,001)	z(0,05)	z(0,10)	z(0,20)	z(0,30)	z(0,40)
0,00	4,086	4,086	4,081	3,782	3,456	2,742	1,939	1,033[b]
0,30	0,072	$-\infty$	-4,009	-0,722	-0,249	0,055	0,072	0,002[c]

D3S20 vs RBP1

Θ_{max}	Z_{max}	z(0,00)	z(0,001)	z(0,05)	z(0,10)	z(0,20)	z(0,30)	z(0,40)
0,00	5,243	5,243	5,234	4,753	4,240	3,161	2,045	0,971[b]
0,00	1,733	1,733	1,729	1,532	1,326	0,897	0,466	0,112[c]
0,00	6,976	6,976	6,963	6,285	5,566	4,058	2,511	1,083[d]

[a]Symbols: Θ_{max}=best estimate for the recombination frequency (Θ); z_{max}=lod score (z) for that recombination fraction

[b,c,d]Data from pedigree 20, family S., and sum, respectively

ACKNOWLEDGMENTS

This study has been financially supported by the Deutsche Forschungsgemeinschaft, the Meyer-Schwarting Stiftung (Bremen), the Deutsche Retinitis Pigmentosa Vereinigung (Karben), and the British Retinitis Pigmentosa Society. We are grateful to Dr. Frank Halliday and Ms Lee Adams of the Retinal Dystrophy Service at the Prince of Wales Hospital, Sydney, and Dr. Pamela Dickinson of the Victorian Eye and Ear Hospital, Melbourne for providing clinical information on these pedigrees. A. Gal is the recipient of a Hermann und Lilly Schilling professorship.

REFERENCES

1. Heckenlively, J.R., *Retinitis pigmentosa*, Lippincott, Philadelphia, 1988.

2. Dryja, T.P., McGee, T.L., Reichel, E., Hahn, L.B., Cowley, G.S., Yandell, D.W., Sandberg, M.A., and Berson,E.L., A point mutation of the rhodopsin gene in one form of retinitis pigmentosa, *Nature*, 343, 364, 1990.

3. Naylor, S.L. and Bishop, D.T., Report of the commit tee on the genetic constitution of chromosome 3. 10th Human Gene Mapping Workshop (HGM10), *Cytogenet. Cell Genet.*, 51, 106, 1989.

4. McWilliam, P., Farrar, G.J., Kenna, P., Bradley, D.G., Humphries, M.M., Sharp, E.M., McConnell, D.J., Lawler, M., Sheils, D., Ryan, C., Stevens, K., Daiger, S.P., and Humphries, P., Autosomal dominant retinitis pigmentosa (ADRP): Localization of an ADRP gene to the long arm of chromosome 3, *Genomics*, 5, 619, 1989.

5. Farrar, G.J., McWilliam, P., Bradley, D.G., Kenna, P., Sharp, E.M., Humphries, M.M., Lawler, M., Eiberg, H., Heckenlively, J.R., Conneally, M.P., Trofatter, J.A., Daiger, S.P., and Humphries, P., Dominant retinitis pigmentosa: Linkage to rhodopsin and evidence for genetic heterogeneity, *Genomics*, in press.

6. Olsson, J.E., Samanns, Ch., Jimenez, J., Pongratz, J., Chand, A., Watty, A., Seuchter, S.A., Denton, M., and Gal, A., Gene of type II autosomal dominant retinitis pigmentosa maps on the long arm of chromosome 3, *Am. J. Med. Genet.*, 35, 595, 1990.

7. Watty, A., Olsson, J.E., Samanns, Ch., Denton, M., and Gal, A., unpublished data, 1990.

8. Chand, A., Olsson, J.E., Adams, L., and Denton, M.J., Exclusion of the autosomal dominant retinitis pigmentosa gene from a substantial region of chromosome 1: study of a large Australian family, *Aust. NZ. J.*

Ophthalmol., 18, 163, 1990.

9. Massof, R.W. and Finkelstein, D., Two forms of autosomal dominant primary retinitis pigmentosa, *Doc.
   Ophthalmol.*, 51, 289, 1981.

10. Fishman, G.A., Alexander, K.R., and Anderson, R.J.,
    Autosomal dominant retinitis pigmentosa. A method of
    classification, *Arch. Ophthalmol.*, 103, 366, 1985.

11. Denton, M.J., Chen, J.D., Serravalle, S., Colley, P.,
    Halliday, F.B., and Donald, J., Analysis of the lin-
    kage relationship of X-linked retinitis pigmentosa
    with the following Xp loci: L1.28, OTC, 754, XJ1.1,
    pERT 87, and C7. *Hum. Genet.*, 78, 60, 1984.

12. Gal, A., Mücke, J., Theile, H., Wieacker, P.F.,
    Ropers, H.H., and Wienker, T.F., X-linked dominant
    Charcot-Marie-Tooth disease: Suggestion of linkage
    with a cloned DNA sequence from the proximal Xq, *Hum.
    Genet.*,70, 38, 1985.

13. Colantuoni, V., Cortese, R., Nilsson, M., Lundvall,
    J., Bavik, C.O., Eriksson, U., Peterson, P.A., and
    Sundelin, J., Cloning and sequencing of a full length
    cDNA corresponding to human cellular retinol-binding
    protein, *Biochem. Biophys. Res. Comm.*, 130, 431,
    1985.

14. Rocchi, M., Covone, A., Romeo, G., Faraonio, R., and
    Colantuoni, V., Regional mapping of RBP4 to 10q23-q24
    and RBP1 to 3q21-q22 in man, *Somatic Cell Mol. Ge
    net.*, 15, 185, 1989.

15. Pellegrino, A., Garofalo, S., Cocozza, S., Monti
    celli, A., Faraonio, R., Varrone, S., and Colantuoni,
    V., TaqI RFLP in the human cellular retinol-binding
    protein (CRBP) gene, *Nucl. Acids Res.*, 16, 15, 7758,
    1988.

16. Ott, J., Estimation of the recombination fraction in
    human pedigrees: Efficient computation of the likeli-
    hood for human linkage studies, *Am. J. Hum. Genet.*,
    26, 588, 1974.

17. Bhattacharya, S.S., personal communication, 1990

REFSUM'S SYNDROME-HEREDOPATHIA ATACTICA POLYNEURITIFORMIS CONCEPTS FOR THERAPY

Dr.F.B.Gibberd M.D.,F.R.C.P.
Consultant Neurologist
Westminster Hospital, London SW1P 2AP, U.K.

1.INTRODUCTION

About forty five years ago Heredopathia Atactica Polyneuritiformis was first described in families in Norway by Refsum.[1] The patients had retinitis pigmentosa, neuropathy, bone deformities and various other abnormalities. Subsequently many other cases have been described and the condition became better known as Refsum's disease. In 1963 Heredopathia Atactica Polyneuritiformis was found to be associated with a raised phytanic acid level in the blood and tissues.[2] It was then discovered that some manifestations of the disease could be helped by lowering the phytanic acid level in the blood either by dietary restriction or by plasma exchange. The disease is inherited as an autosomal recessive.

2.BIOCHEMISTRY OF PHYTANIC ACID

Phytanic Acid has the following formula:

$$CH_3-CH(CH_3)-CH_2-CH_2-CH_2-CH(CH_3)-CH_2-CH_2-CH(CH_3)-CH_2-CH_2-CH(CH_3)-CH_2-CH_2-COOH$$

The unusual aspect of this aliphatic carboxylic acid is the presence of methyl side chains which are not found in other fatty acids. Phytanic acid is derived from phytol by oxidation and then hydrogenation.

CH3   CH3   CH3   CH3   H

CH   CH2   CH   CH2   CH   CH2   C   CHOH   PHYTOL

CH3 CH2 CH2 CH2 CH2 CH2 CH2 CH

Most long chain fatty acids are broken down by beta-oxidation when two carbon moieties are removed at a time from the carboxylic end of the molecule so that carbons alpha and beta are removed together

CH2   *CH2:   COOH

CH2   :CH2

Beta:Oxidation

Because phytanic acid has a methyl group on the gamma carbon(*) beta oxidation is not possible and an initial alpha oxidation is necessary before beta oxidation can break down the rest of the fatty acid chain

CH3

CH2   *CH   ;COOH

CH2   CH2 :

Alpha:Oxidation

Alpha oxidation is needed only for the metabolism of phytanic acid as there are no other fatty acids with methyl groups in similar positions; patients with Heredopathia Atactica Polyneuritiformis lack the enzyme required for alpha oxidation so that phytanic acid accumulates in their bodies. A small amount of fatty acids can be slowly metabolised from the omega carbon by omega oxidation

: CH3

: CH2

CH3 :   CH2

Omega:Oxidation

In normal people omega oxidation is so insignificant that it cannot be detected easily but in patients with Heredopathia Atactica Polyneuritiformis in whom there is no other way of removing it about 10mg(32micromols) of phytanic acid can be removed daily by this process. The metabolism from the omega end of the molecule cannot proceed to complete breakdown but stops when methyladipic acid which can be detected in the urine is formed. [3]

CH3 CH2 CH COOH HOOC CH2 CH2   METHYLADIPIC ACID

3.CLINICAL

The clinical manifestations of Heredopathia Atactica Polyneuritiformis can be considered under three headings. [4]

A.SKELETAL ABNORMALITIES

Skeletal changes are noted in about a third of patients. They are present when the disease is first diagnosed and they are possibly congenital although they have never been demonstrated at birth. This could be due to the fact that Heredopathia Atactica Polyneuritiformis has never been diagnosed at birth or because the skeletal changes develop during bone formation. The commonest easily-noted change is a shortening of the terminal phalanx of the thumb although other fingers may be involved less obviously. Also frequently seen is shortening of one or more of the metacarpal or metatarsal bones. The changes are not always symmetrical. The reason for the bone changes is not known. It may be that the absence of the enzyme for alpha-oxidation or the excess phytanic acid leads to an abnormality of bone when it is being laid down. Alternatively the condition may be associated with a separate disease of bone, with the two genes being close together on the same chromosome.

B.DEGENERATION IN SPECIAL SENSE ORGANS

The most widely recognised of the abnormalities in Heredopathia Atactica Polyneuritiformis is retinitis pigmentosa. This usually presents as night blindness in childhood or adolescence, although frequently the condition is not recognised until adult life. The retinitis pigmentosa develops very slowly and it has not been observed to progress in patients on a therapeutic diet. There are frequently cataracts which may develop in the third decade and are progressive despite a therapeutic diet. The cataracts which are frequently associated with a small pupil are often a greater handicap than the retinitis pigmentosa.

Although less often recognised loss of the sense of smell is characteristic. As this symptom is not often associated with other genetic, metabolic, neurological and ophthalmological diseases it is an important symptom and sign in assessing whether a patient with retinitis pigmentosa may have Heredopathia Atactica Polyneuritiformis. The loss of smell may be present before the retinitis pigmentosa and may occur so early in life that the patient does not know what normal smell is. Therefore it is not adequate just to ask the patient if they can smell: it needs to be tested.

Many patients develop deafness which is sensorineural. This can come on either gradually or suddenly. The deafness of gradual onset comes on later than the retinitis pigmentosa and is unlikely to be improved by therapeutic diet although progression may cease. However during acute exacerbations of the disease, deafness may become rapidly worse over a period of weeks. This sudden deterioration is reversible with therapy.

C.ACUTE MANIFESTATIONS

There are a number of clinical manifestations that are closely linked to the level of phytanic acid in the blood. When the level rises the manifestations develop over a period of weeks but can rapidly worsen in days. All these manifestations improve and usually clear completely when the phytanic acid level falls. The most important of these findings is a peripheral neuropathy which can be so bad that a patient is unable to walk or feed himself. In addition the patient may have ichthyosis, cardiac arrythmias, cardiomyopathy, myopathy and severe anorexia.

4.PRINCIPLES OF MANAGEMENT

The evidence is that phytanic acid in the blood is the toxic agent; this is definite for the acute manifestations, although it has not been proved for the bony abnormalities and the degeneration in the special sense organs. This could be because the diet has never been given before the bones and sense organs are affected and the irreversible damage in these organs could not be helped by reducing the phytanic acid levels. However the absence of progression in the damage to the retina and hearing after therapy suggests that the phytanic acid level in the body is important. Therefore the first principle of management is to lower the amount of phytanic acid in the body.

There is considerable evidence that the phytanic acid in the fat depots is not toxic, whereas that in the blood is. The evidence for this is that phytanic acid levels in the fat do not correlate with the clinical status but there is a close correlation with the level of phytanic acid in the blood. Also if a patient loses weight for any reason (usually loss of appetite) the blood level of phytanic acid rises and the patient develops an increase in the acute symptoms. The rise in the blood level with starvation is due to the fact that as body fat is utilised for energy purposes all the fatty acids are metabolised except phytanic acid, the concentration of which therefore rises in the blood. Conversely the acute symptoms are improved if a patient eats well and puts on weight. In these circumstances the phytanic acid is taken out of the blood and put into the fat depots. The second principle of management is to lower the blood level of phytanic acid in acute illness, even if the total body phytanic acid is not altered.

One can therefore draw up a diagramatic picture of the dynamic changes which are occuring in the body of a patient with Heredopathia Atactica Polyneuritiformis showing the various ways in which phytanic acid is metabolised and can be removed. By utilising the possible pathways the patient can be treated.

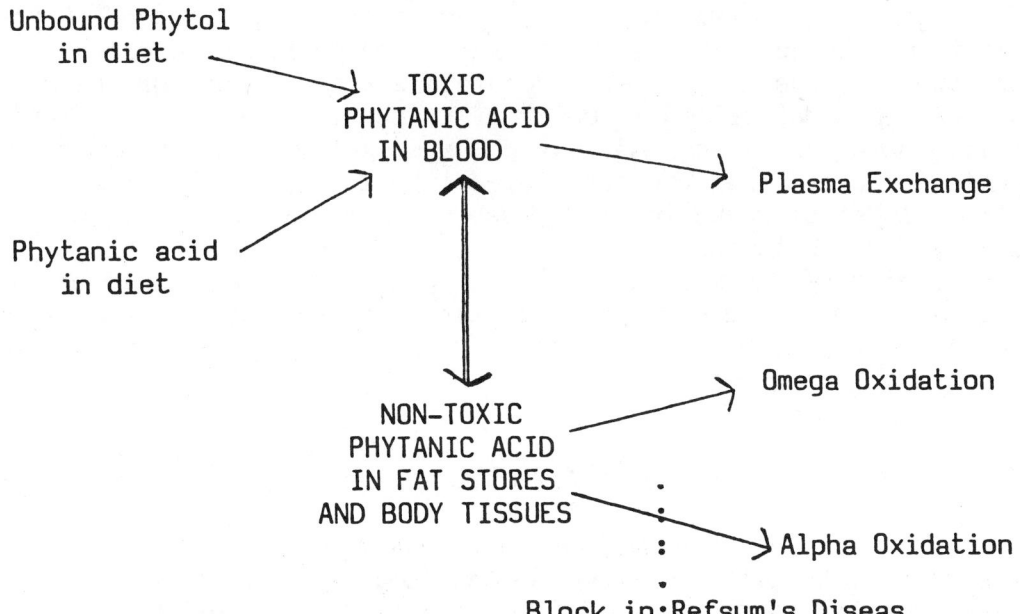

```
Unbound Phytol
   in diet
                    →  TOXIC
                    PHYTANIC ACID
                       IN BLOOD  ───────→   Plasma Exchange

Phytanic acid
   in diet


                    NON-TOXIC          →  Omega Oxidation
                   PHYTANIC ACID
                   IN FAT STORES   .
                  AND BODY TISSUES  :
                                    :  →  Alpha Oxidation
                                    .
                    Block in:Refsum's Diseas
```

Relevant amounts of phytanic acid in micromols: [5]

Average daily intake in Europeans:	160
P.A. removable in one plasma exchange:	up to 4,800
Maximum omega oxidation per day:	32

Phytanic acid in blood in micromols/litre

Normal person:	0-33
An untreated patient with Refsum's disease:	950-6400
A treated patient with Refsum's disease:	16-704

5.PLASMA EXCHANGE

As phytanic acid is present in the lipid fractions of the plasma, plasma exchange is an efficient method of removing it. Plasma exchange removes the phytanic acid from that compartment of the body from whence it does the most harm. A large amount can be removed at one session. However it is an invasive procedure and has serious risks. There are the risks run in any plasma exchange when foreign proteins are introduced and immune reactions can occur. This is more likely to occur if plasma exchange is used on many occasions. Also plasma exchange places considerable stress on the cardiovascular system at a time when patients ill with Heredopathia Atactica Polyneuritiformis, may have cardiac abnormalities with arrythmias and poor cardiac function. Therefore it should be used with caution. However, as the amount of phytanic acid removed is considerable, the treatment is particularly helpful when a patient is very ill. Acutely ill patients have anorexia and find it difficult to take a diet which will cause them to put on weight. Plasma exchange is usually carried out three times over a period of about a fortnight. The maximum amount of phytanic acid is removed at the first procedure, at the end of which the phytanic acid level in the blood may be quite low. Therefore a second procedure carried out within a day or two is unlikely to remove much more phytanic acid. However if one waits about a week there is a passage of phytanic acid from the fat stores into the blood so that the blood level of phytanic acid rises and further plasma exchanges remove more phytanic acid.

Therefore the main indications for using plasma exchange are rapidly progressing disease, arrhythmias which might cause sudden death, severe cachexia and failure to respond to the diet.

6.PHYTOL

Phytanic acid is derived from phytol which is a part of the chlorophyll complex in green plants. Most dietary phytol is bound in chlorophyll and not easily absorbed by man so that most green foods can be eaten by patients with Heredopathia Atactica Polyneuritiformis.[6] However when phytol is free it is absorbed and rapidly converted into phytanic acid. In a normal person this phytanic acid is quickly metabolised, but in patients with Heredopathia Atactica Polyneuritiformis it accumulates.

What is more important is that ruminants and other animals which feed largely on green foods have bacteria in their gastrointestinal tracts which free phytol so that both phytol and phytanic acid are efficiently absorbed. Hence the fat of ruminants contains a relatively high level of phytanic acid compared to other animals. If a normal man eats such fat it is easily metabolised but if a patient with Refsum's disease does so the phytanic acid is not metabolised so the concentration in the body rises.

7.DIETARY MANAGEMENT

The principles of dietary management are:
1. Low phytanic acid intake
2. Sufficient calorie intake
3. Palatability
4. Nutritional adequacy

When patients are well, have a good appetite and no cachexia the blood level of phytanic acid will decrease if they adhere to the prescribed diet low in phytanic acid. In these circumstances omega oxidation will remove a significant amount of phytanic acid. However when patients are ill and anorexic they often do not eat sufficient to maintain body weight and further phytanic acid leaves the fat stores and the level in the blood rises. When patients are unwell the diet has to be more strict. Therefore two levels of diet are used.

1. Blood phytanic acid above 320micromols/litre
High calorie diet
Low phytanic acid diet
Attempt to move phytanic acid from blood to fat stores

2. Blood phytanic acid below 320micromols/litre
Low phytanic acid diet
Achieve or maintain normal weight

The diets are divided into different stages.[7,8]

A.STAGE 1

This is a liquid diet and contains no phytanic acid. It can be given by nasogastric tube if the patient is to ill to eat or if anorexia makes eating too distasteful. It is not palatable but is very effective. It can usually be maintained for only a few weeks. As used at Westminster Hospital it consists of:

100g Marvel   135g Caloreen
10ml Safflower seed oil   30ml Crusha
Water to 1 litre to produce:
1016 K Cal, 36.4g protein per litre. No phytanic acid

B.STAGE 2

This consists of the liquid diet with solid foods containing less than 0.5mg(1.6micromols) per 100g of the food. Examples of such foods are: wholemeal bread, eggs, turkey and chicken meat, some margarines, jam, honey and skimmed milk.

C.STAGE 3

This is a much more liberal diet. The liquid diet in stage 1 is abandoned. In addition to taking the foods of the Stage 2 diet, measured amounts of other foods, which contain between 0.5 and 2mg per 100g of the food, are allowed so that the total daily amount of phytanic acid ingested remains below 10mg (32micromols). Such foods are pork, fish, potatoes, beans and cereals. Each food needs to be individually measured. Patients can state their preferences to the dietitian and the particular food assayed. Food containing only a small amount of phytanic acid can be added to the diet. Some foods, such as full cream milk, butter, beef, lamb and foodstuffs derived from these contain large amounts of phytanic acid and therefore are completely excluded. At this stage phytol containing foods are excluded because even the small amount of free phytol absorbed may decrease the effectiveness of the diet.

D.STAGE 4

This is the same as the stage 3 diet with the addition of phytol containing foods. When this diet is used the patient's phytanic acid level in the blood is low so that there is little danger of an acute exacerbation. If the blood level of phytanic acid is monitored it is possible to foretell any potential for deterioration so that the diet can then be made more strict. However allowing the addition of phytol containing foods the diet becomes much more liberal and it is easier for the patient to maintain the diet permanently.

The dietary stage is decided by the patient's clinical condition in association with the blood phytanic acid level. In acutely ill patients Stage 1 is first used, but in mild cases Stage 3 may be commenced initially. In patients who are well and whose blood phytanic acid level is low Stage 4 is used.

8.ACKNOWLEDGEMENTS

I would like to thank the British Retinitis Pigmentosa Society for financial assistance in the research on Refsum's disease.

9. REFERENCES

1. Refsum, S., A familial syndrome not hitherto described. A contribution to the clinical study of the hereditary disorders of the nervous system. Acta Psychiatrica Scandinavica, Supplement 38. 1946

2. Klenk,E. and Kahlke,W. Uber das Vorkommen der 3,7,11,15-Tetramethyl-Hexadecansaure (Phytansaure) in den Cholesterinestern und anderen Lipoidfraktionend der organe bei einem Krankheitsfall undekannter Genese (Verdacht auf Heredopathia Atactica Polyneuritiformis Refsum-like syndrome). Hoppe-seyler Zeitschrift Physiologische Chemie, 333,133, 1963.

3. Krywawych,S.,Brenton,D.P.,Jackson,M.J., Forte,C., Walker,D.K. and Lawson,A.M., Methyladipate excretion in animals fed a phytol supplement with reference to Refum's disease. J.Inher.Metabol.Dis. 30,342,1984.

4. Gibberd,F.B.,Billimoria,J.D.,Goldman,J.M.,Clemens.M.E., Evans,R.,Whitelaw,M.N.,Retsas,S. and Sherratt,R.M., Heredopathia Atactica Polyneuritiformis. Refsum's disease. Acta Neurologica Scand. 72,1,1985.

5.   Britton,T.C.,Gibberd,F.B.,Clemens,M.E.,Billimoria,J.D. and Sidey,M.C., The significance of plasma phytanic acid levels in adults. J.Neurol.Neurosurg and Psych., 52,891,1989

6. Coppack,S.W.,Evans,R.,Gibberd,F.B.,Clemens,M.E.and Billimoria,J.D., Can patients with Refsum's disease safely eat green vegetables ?. Brit.med.J.,296,828,1988.

7. Masters-Thomas,A., Bailes.J.,Billimoria,J.D., Clemens,M.E.,Gibberd,F.B. and Page,N.G.R., Heredopathia Atactica Polyneuritiformis 1.Clinical Features and Dietary Management. J.of Human Nutrition,34,245,1980

8. Masters-Thomas,A., Bailes.J.,Billimoria,J.D., Clemens,M.E.,Gibberd,F.B. and Page,N.G.R., Heredopathia Atactica Polyneuritiformis 2.Estimation of phytanic acid in food. J.of Human Nutrition,34,251,1980

TREATING RETINAL DEGENERATIONS
BY CELL AND/OR GENE TRANSPLANTATION: WHEN AND HOW?

P. Gouras, J. Du, R. Lopez, R. Kwun,
P. Sforza, H. Kjeldbye, A. Avakian, D. Kauffmann

Edward S. Harkness Eye Institute, Columbia University,
New York, New York U.S.A.

INTRODUCTION

There are two major new approaches on the horizon for the treatment of photoreceptor degenerations of the human retina. One is gene therapy; the other is cell transplantation. In this presentation we briefly assess the major problems involved in using these two different approaches. Then we concentrate on where current research, and our laboratory in particular, stand on cell transplantation therapy.

Gene therapy depends upon a number of factors. Most important, it is necessary to know the gene or genes that are defective. For most of the retinal degenerations this is not yet known but this drawback is gradually being eliminated. Another and more serious problem in using this approach is that the photoreceptors must still be present. If all, or most, of the photoreceptors have degenerated then there is little value in gene therapy because it is impossible to insert genes into cells that are no longer there. Many of the retinal degenerations we face in the clinic do involve the loss of many or most of the photoreceptors. A third problem with gene therapy in the central nervous system in general, and in the retina in particular, is that cells like photoreceptors, retinal epithelium and Muller cells, all of which may be involved in these diseases, are non-replicating cells. This makes it more difficult to use retrovirus vectors to introduce foreign genes into cells. More radical and therefore less predictable methods must be resorted to such as the use of neurotropic viruses as vectors such as rabies or herpes virus.[1] Therefore there are some significant problems associated with gene therapy. This approach has its best chance to help when applied at a relatively early stage in any retinal degeneration before most of the photoreceptors have degenerated.

On the other hand cell transplantation is best designed to treat those diseases where all or most of the photoreceptors have degenerated and consequently are absent in the area where the transplanted cells would go. Cell transplantation has completely different problems. A major hurdle for cell transplantation is whether the microsurgical techniques can be developed to place foreign cells in the appropriate place in the retina and guarantee their long term survival. In the case of photoreceptors an additional requirement is needed. Each cell, preferably the cones, must form synapses with appropriate second order neurons. Host/graft rejection, a recurrent problem with all types of allografts is less problematic with the advent of powerful immunosuppressant drugs, some of which may be effective if applied locally within the eye. In addition the retina, being in the central nervous system, may be an immunologically privileged site. Cell transplantation could of course treat non-genetic degenerations of the photoreceptors as sometimes occur from drug toxicity or bacterial or viral infections.

Retinal Epithelial Cell Transplantation

    In our own laboratory we have been developing techniques to transplant retinal epithelium and/or photoreceptors to the retina of animal models with retinal dystrophies. We started this approach with retinal epithelial cells because these cells seemed the most tractable.[2-4] The first experiments designed to alter a hereditary retinal degeneration were performed on Royal College of Surgeons (RCS) strain of rats because the defect is known to be due to a failure of the retinal epithelium to phagocytize the effete tips of the growing outer segments. We thought that since transplanted retinal epithelial cells were able to phagocytize host outer segments[4] we should be able to restore this function in the RCS rat retina and thereby correct the genetic defect. In order to transplant retinal epithelium into the rat retina by an anterior approach we had to modify our surgical technique to avoid the relatively large rat lens. We succeeded with this in late 1987.[5] This very exciting experiment was appreciated by another laboratory who had now entered the field by following our progress with retinal epithelial cell transplantation. They employed a posterior approach through the choroid which requires more touch than sight. Both laboratories reached the same conclusion at the same time.[6,7] There was a striking preservation in photoreceptor survival following retinal epithelial cell transplantation. Figure 1 (next page) shows examples of this saving of photoreceptors. Figure 1A shows the retina of a normal rat. Figure 1B shows the retina of an RCS rat at 4 months of age; all of the photoreceptors have disappeared leading to a neural retina that is about half the normal thickness. Figure 1 C and D show retinas of two different RCS rats, 5 months old, but which had received retinal epithelial cell transplants at infancy (15-18 days of age). There is a striking preservation of photoreceptors, including not only the nuclei but the inner and outer segments. The transplanted retinal epithelial cells can be identified by their pigmentation. This is a most remarkable phenomenon and represents the first time that any hereditary disease of the central nervous system has been successfully treated by cell transplantation. This success has been an enormous stimulus for further research on cell transplantation in all animal models of retinal degenerations.

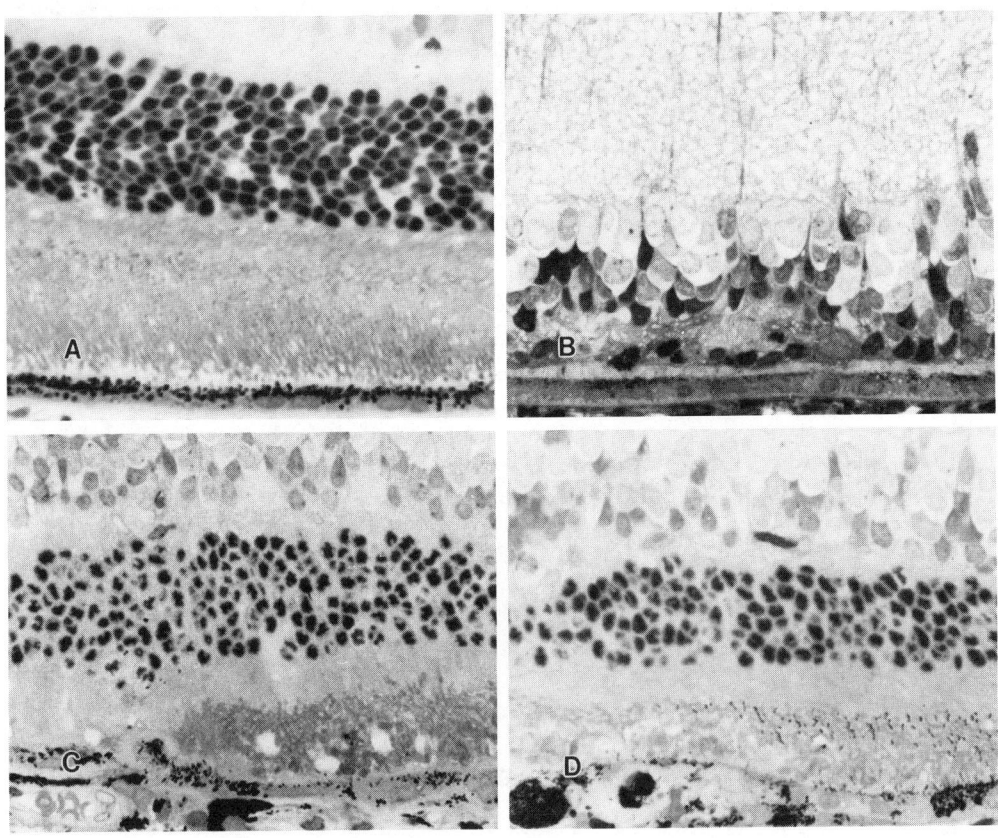

Figure 1. Light micrographs from a four month old normal pigmented (A), tan hooded RCS dystrophic (B), and from RCS dystrophic rats that have received transplanted normal retinal epithelium four months previously (C,D). Magnification is 140X

The Cause of the Photoreceptor Rescue

From the beginning we have noticed that as soon as the transplanted epithelial cells are placed in the subretinal space they begin to phagocytize outer segment material voraciously.[7] Therefore phagocytosis of outer segments, the basic defect in this dystrophy, is corrected immediately. Figure 2 (next page) illustrates the status of pigmented retinal epithelial cells transplanted to the subretinal space of RCS rat retina four months previously. The pigmented cells are normal in ultrastructural appearance; some appear to be actively synthesizing melanin (closed arrows); fresh phagosomal material is present in their cytoplasm (open arrows) indicating that they are still performing this important aspect of their function in the dystrophic rat retina. It is interesting that the transplant cells are lying on top of the albinotic host epithelium.

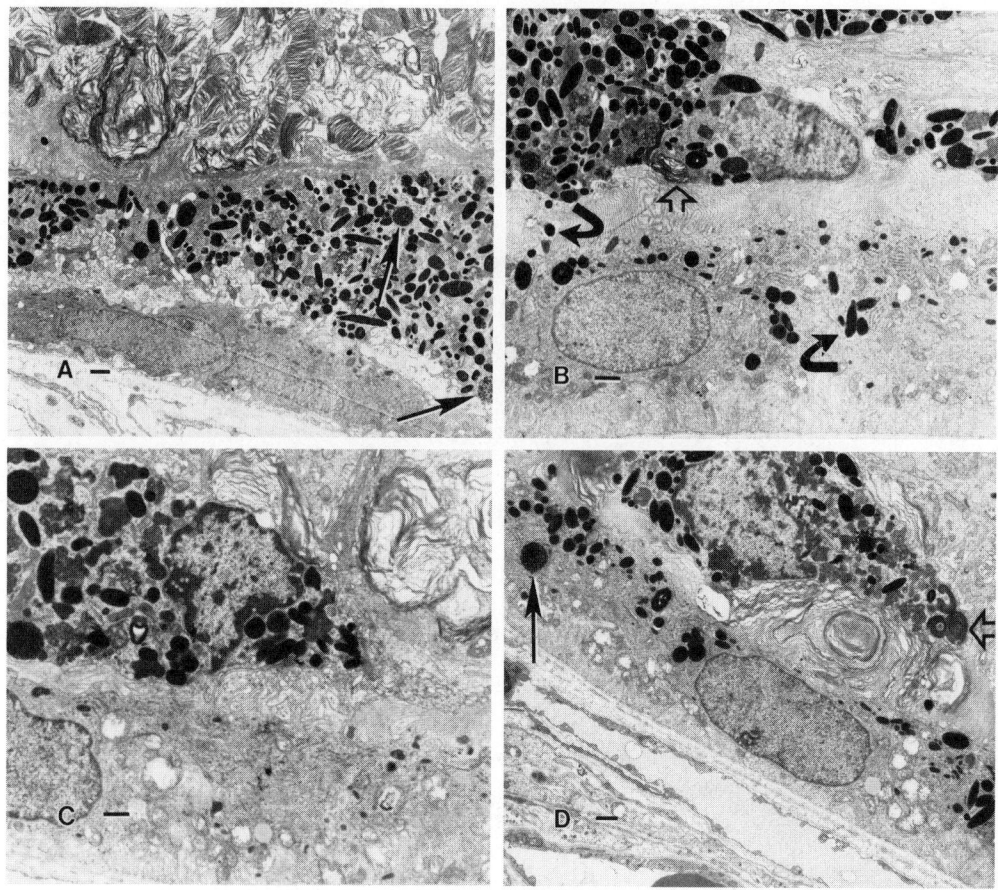

Figure 2. Electron micrographs of transplanted retinal epithelial cells next to host cells which are on Bruch's membrane. The transplant cells are filled with lysosomal material and melanin granules. Phagosomes can also be seen and are indicated by the open arrows. Curved arrows point out a series of melanin granules and straight arrows premelanosomes. The bars indicate 1 micron.

Figure 3 (next page) shows a relationship between the number of transplant cells and the amount of photoreceptors rescued within a local area of the RCS rat retina. The greater the number of transplant cells, the greater is the rescue of neighboring photoreceptors. There is therefore a link between the presence of a transplant cell and photoreceptor survival. There is, however, some survival of photoreceptors in areas where no transplant cell can be found. We began to notice this the more we quantitated photoreceptor survival from transplantation and mentioned this in an editorial in 1989.[8]

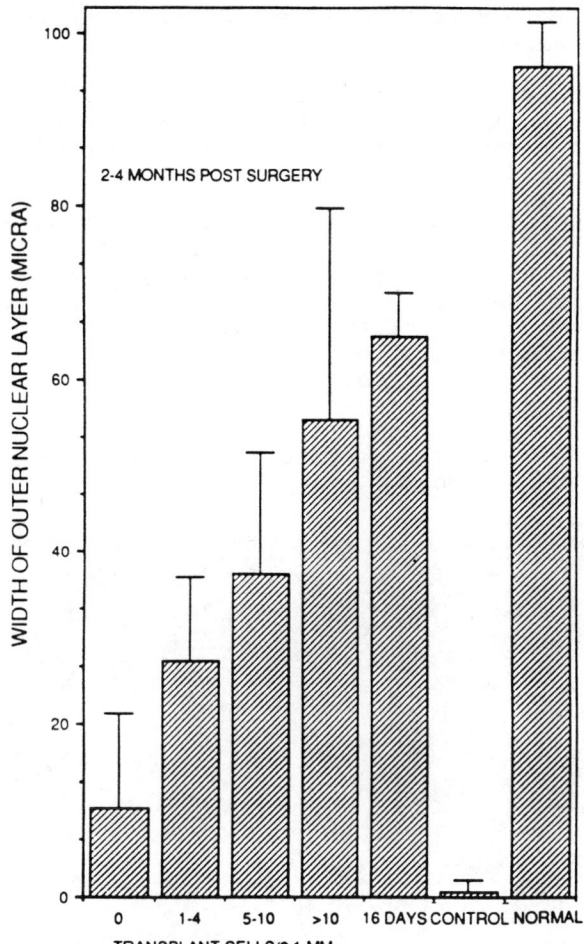

2-4 MONTHS POST SURGERY

WIDTH OF OUTER NUCLEAR LAYER (MICRA)

TRANSPLANT CELLS/0.1 MM

Figure 3. Histogram of measurements obtained through the area of the retina of 5 dystrophic rats that had received transplant 2-4 months previously, through un-operated eyes (control) of these rats and through a similar area of a 16 day old dystrophic rat, which is at or just before the surgery was performed on the other 5 dystrophic rats. Measurements of a normal rat of 5 months of age is shown on the far right.

Recently several other laboratories have reported that photoreceptors can be rescued in the RCS retina without transplanting retinal epithelium.[9,10] This conflicts but is not incompatible with the idea that it is the restoration of phagocytosis that is responsible for stopping the retinal degeneration (see below). We have also examined sham surgery including saline injections, mechanical damage, external diathermy and transplantation of dystrophic retinal epithelium. We find that these procedures produce a different effect than normal epithelial cell transplants in the following ways:

1) It tends to be localized to the area where the procedure is performed; normal retinal epithelial cell transplants produce saving over a larger area following their diffusion into the subretinal space.

2) It is not as effective; it is rare to find any outer segments surviving by sham procedures alone.

3) It is not as long lasting; we have receptor survival at 15 months after retinal epithelial cell transplants whereas it has been difficult to obtain significant survival after 4-5 months from the sham procedure.

We have found that all surgical procedures attract macrophages into the subretinal space. These macrophages are also capable of phagocytizing outer segments. Figure 4 shows a macrophage that has entered the subretinal space by retinal surgery. It is also filled with fresh phagosomes. Therefore some of the effects on photoreceptor survival from sham surgery could be due to macrophage phagocytosis of outer segments. Whether this is the complete explanation is not established but it is a very viable hypothesis. What this interesting controversy has shown is that a technique designed to treat a particular retinal degeneration is casting new light on the pathogenesis of this disease.

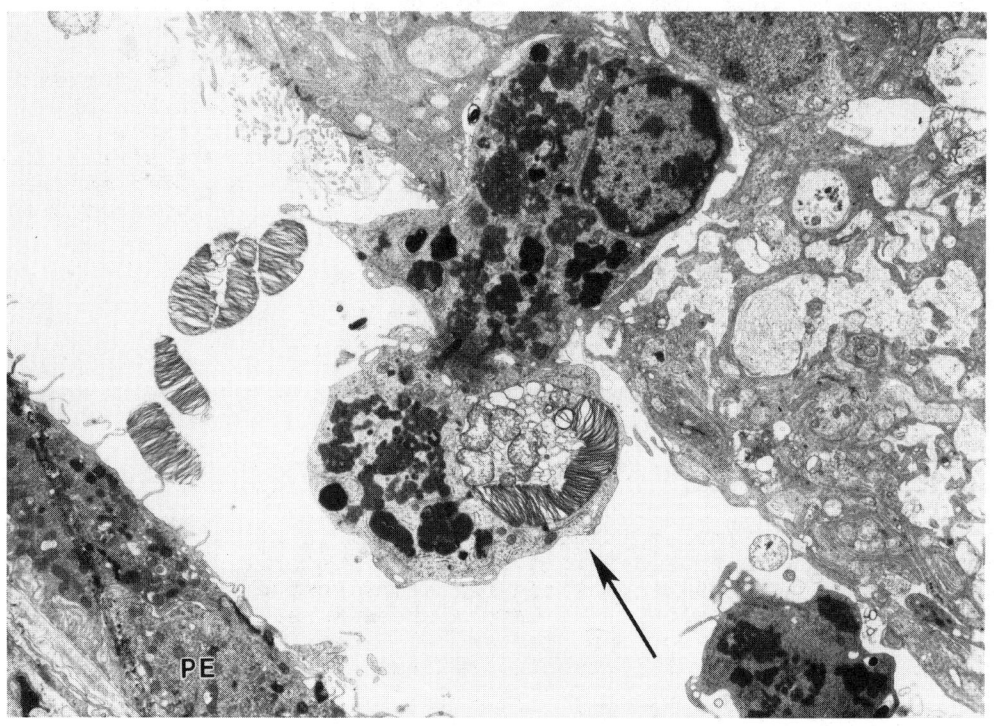

Figure 4. Electron micrograph of a macrophage penetrating the retina 30 minutes after subretinal surgery. The macrophage is filled with lysosomes and has already incorporated outer segment material (arrow).

Photoreceptor Transplants

Our experience with the RCS rat led us to ask whether we could use transplantation techniques to treat the adult stage of this disease when virtually all the photoreceptor cells have degenerated. This is a stage of retinal degeneration which is no longer amenable to gene therapy. It mimics, however, many of the patients we encounter with Retinitis Pigmentosa. Our strategy was to transplant <u>both</u> normal photoreceptors and retinal epithelial cells to the subretinal space of the adult (4-5 month old) RCS rat.

In order to label the transplanted photoreceptors we injected newborn normal rats with ^{3}H-thymidine each day for a week. This labeled at least 50% of the photoreceptors. This was determined by injecting dissociated photoreceptors obtained from these radiolabeled rats into the vitreous of a donor rat; we examined these vitreal cells by autoradiography. Figure 5A shows a toluidine blue stained section and 5B the adjacent section by autoradiography. The ratio of the number of labeled nuclei to total nuclei is 0.49, a value consistent with the number of dividing postnatal rods in the rat.[11]

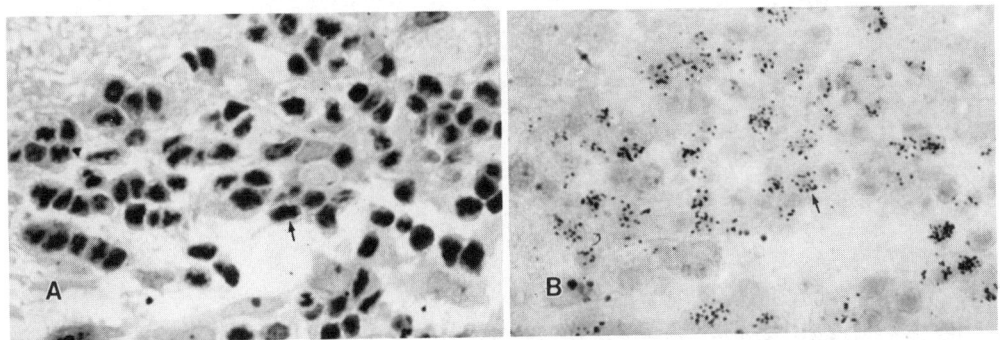

Figure 5. **A.** Light photomicrograph of rat photoreceptors transplanted to the vitreous of a host rat 7 days previously. The receptor (arrow) cells are organized into a cluster abutting the inner limiting membrane of the retina. Photoreceptor nuclei of rods in particular have a characteristic clumped chromatin staining pattern to their nucleus.

B. Autoradiograph of a section close to the one shown in Figure 5A. Many of the nuclei have clusters of grains (arrow) produced by radiation from tritiated thymidine contained in the nuclei of the transplanted rods.

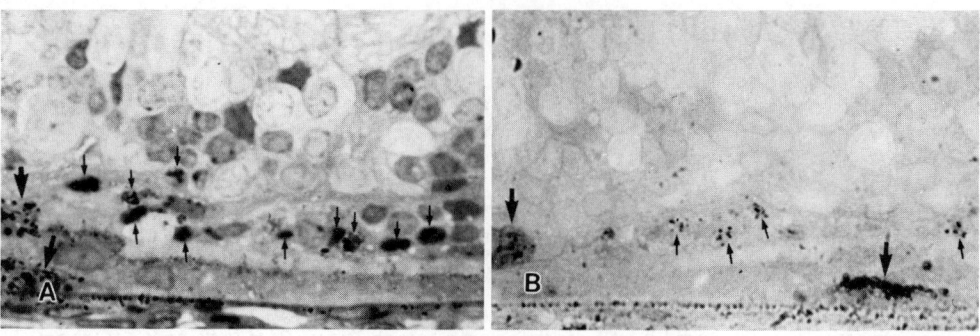

Figure 6. **A.** Light photomicrograph of a retina from a 5 month old RCS rat which received transplanted photoreceptors and pigmented retinal epithelial cells 14 days previously. The darkly staining nuclei in an area corresponding to the external nuclear layer, are transplanted photoreceptors (small arrows). The cells with dark granules on the lower left are co-transplanted pigmented retinal epithelial cells (large arrows).

B. Autoradiograph of a section close to that shown in Figure 6A. There are four distinctly labeled nuclei (small arrows) in the same region where the putative rod nuclei are seen in Figure 6A. Transplanted pigmented retinal epithelial cells are also visible at the lower left and right of this section (large arrows).

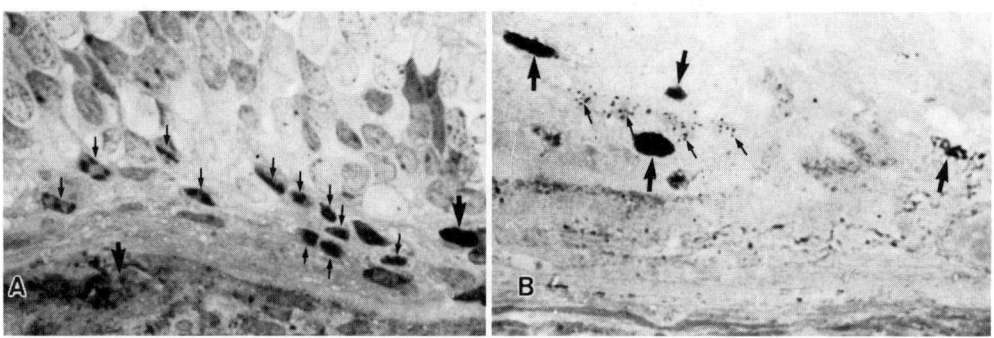

Figure 7. **A.** Light photomicrograph of a retina from a 5 month old RCS rat which received transplanted photoreceptors and pigment retinal epithelial cells 30 days previously. The cluster of darkly staining nuclei in an area corresponding to the external nuclear layer, are transplanted photoreceptors (small arrows). Transplanted, pigmented epithelial cells are also seen in this section (large arrows).

B. Autoradiograph of a section close to that shown in Figure 7A. There are four distinctly, labeled nuclei (small arrow) in the same region where the putative rod nuclei are seen in Figure 7A. Pigmented retinal epithelial cells surround the transplanted photoreceptors (large arrows).

Figures 6 and 7 (previous page) show transplanted rod nuclei demonstrated by autoradiography at 2 weeks and one month after transplantation. There is therefore no doubt that photoreceptors can survive for a considerable time in the host retina. We now have evidence that photoreceptors survive for at least three months in a host rat. They are, however, not as viable as transplanted pigmented retinal epithelium. We transplant approximately ten times as many photoreceptors as retinal epithelial cells. When we determine the ratio of photoreceptors to pigmented epithelial cells we have found that this ratio is progressively decreasing at 1, 2 and 3 months after transplantation. Since the retinal epithelial cells seem to remain stable for a year after transplantation, there must be a slow attrition of transplanted photoreceptors after they have been transplanted to the subretinal space.

The photoreceptors (rods) that survive appear to make synaptic contacts with the host retinal cells (Figures 8 and 9). We consider this to be a very important phenomenon. Evidence has been presented from three different laboratories that such synapses are occurring.[12-14] All of the evidence is indirect and requires a more unequivocal demonstration that this is correct because it is

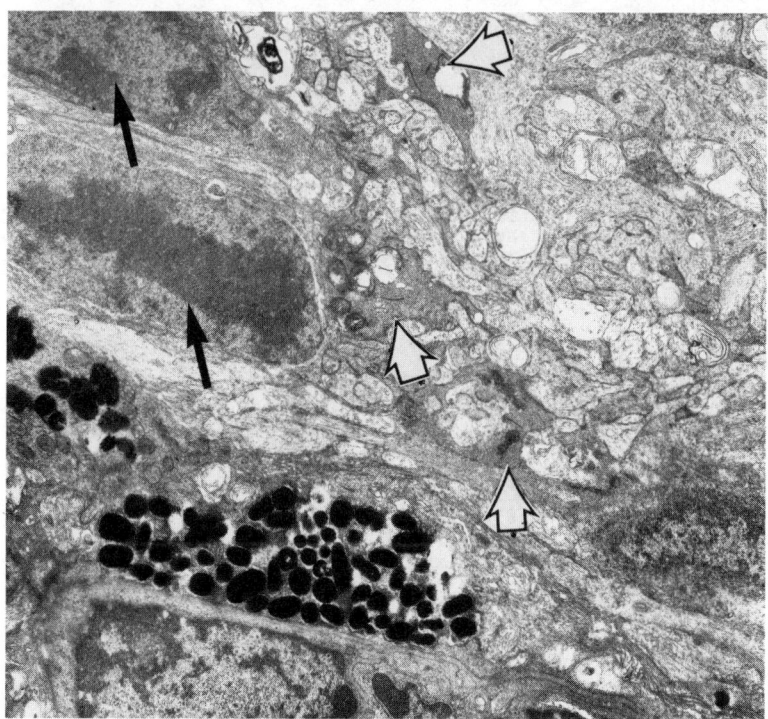

Figure 8. Electron micrograph showing the nuclei of transplanted rods (closed arrows) which have been identified by autoradiography one month after transplantation. Note also the presence of transplanted pigmented retinal epithelial cells which also mark the transplant site. Synaptic vesicles, synaptic ribbons can be seen in the cytoplasm of these rods (open arrows). Magnification 5000X.

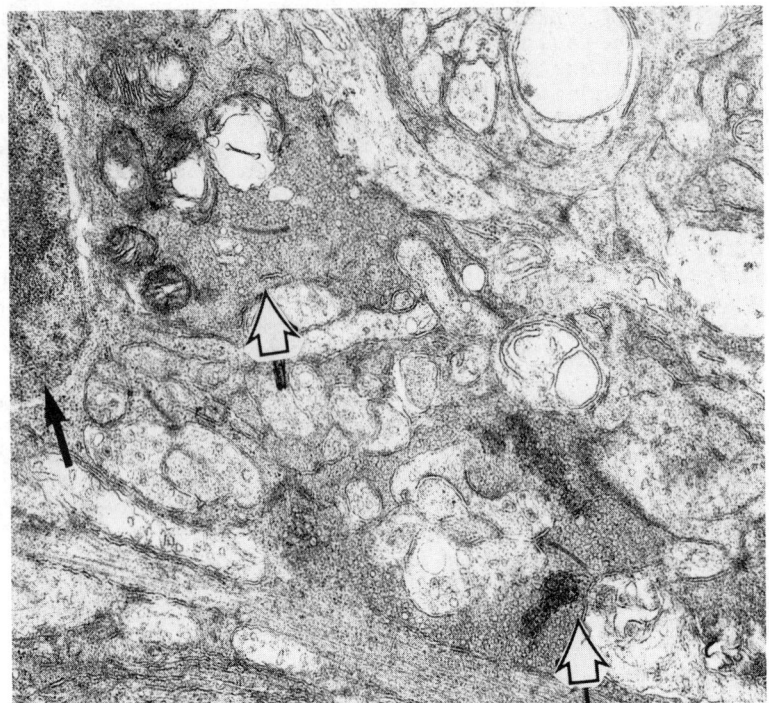

Figure 9. Higher power electron micrograph of the synapses shown in Figure 8 (open arrows). At this magnification pre- and post-synaptic densities can be visualized in some of these synapses. A rod nucleus is also indicated by the filled arrow. Magnification is 20,000X.

so critical for the future of this approach. The evidence from our own lab is the following. In areas where we find transplanted photoreceptors, there is relatively high density of rod spherules containing abundant synaptic vesicles, synaptic ribbons and forming presynaptic densities with other retinal cells. The rod nuclei that are labeled by autoradiography can be examined by electron microscopy from serial sections and within the cytoplasm of these rods we find synapses (Figures 8 and 9). We do not believe these post synaptic cells have come from the donor animal because our enzymatic dissection removes such contacts and examination of our transplant material does not reveal any post synaptic cells. Such a concentration of synapses are not found elsewhere in this or the control retina from the contralateral eye of the rat. There is also evidence from deoxyglucose staining that these photoreceptor transplants may be functional[13] but even this is indirect since such activity could be produced by non-synaptic mechanisms. It will be of great importance to obtain as much evidence as possible that transplanted photoreceptors, which are central nervous system neurons, are capable of reforming synapses with foreign retinal cells. If this hypothesis is correct, then a major hurdle to microsurgical reconstruction of the outer layers of the retina has been overcome.

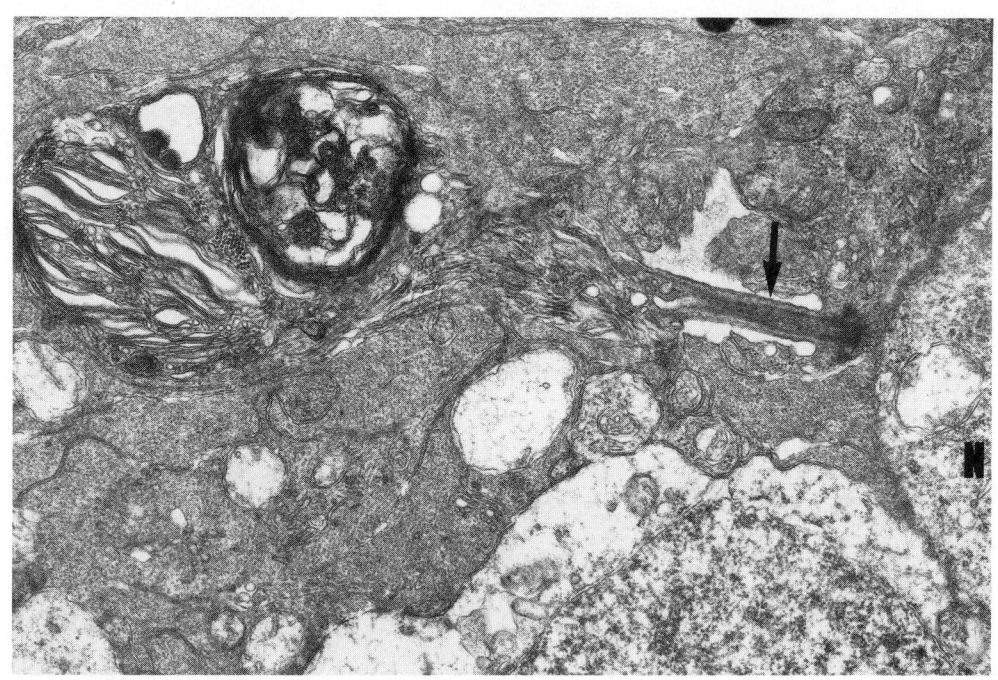

Figure 10. Electron micrograph of a transplanted rod, one month after transplantation. There is a rudimentary outer segment connected to a cilium (arrow). The nucleus (N) of this rod is also visible. Magnification is 20,000X.

The second problem we experience with photoreceptor transplantation is the preservation of the photoreceptive organelle of the cell, the outer segment. Outer segment material becomes very scarce after one month in the host retina. Figure 10 shows how one of these small outer segments appear in a transplanted rod. There is cilium connecting the cell body of the rod to the outer segment, which is, however, only rudimentary in size. We are not yet sure of what the cause of the atrophy of the outer segment is. We have noticed that when we do see an outer segment it is often in close proximity to a normal co-transplanted retinal epithelial cell. Perhaps it will be necessary to pay more attention to aligning the outer segments with either the host or the co-transplanted retinal epithelium in order to insure the outer segment's long term viability. In this sense the RCS rat model may not be ideal because the host retinal epithelium is defective. To this end we have begun transplanting mouse photoreceptors into the C3H mouse retina, in which the genetic defect occurs within the photoreceptor rather than the epithelial cell.

Another explanation for the rudimentary size of the outer segments in the transplanted rods is that the extremely large size of this organelle and its delicate connection to the cell body by a thin cilium leads to its breaking off during the surgical manipulations. To this end we have been experimenting with the transplantation of neonatal photoreceptors which have outer segments which are just making their appearance and consequently less likely to disconnect during transplantation surgery.

Transplantation of Transgenic Cells

In order to identify transplanted cells, especially photoreceptors, at the electron microscopic level we have been using transgenic donor cells in which the bacterial lac-Z gene has been inserted into the genome of retinal epithelial cells or rods. The latter transgenic rods have been produced by Jeremy Nathans, who has inserted the rhodopsin promoter coupled to the lac-Z gene into the germline of a mouse strain. The rods of these mice express the bacterial galactosidase, which is stainable by histochemical techniques both at the light and electron microscopic level. This may provide a more definitive demonstration of synapse formation by transplanted rods at the electron microscopic level.

The rat retinal epithelial cells have been made transgenic by inserting the lac-Z gene into their genome while they are in culture. Success with gene expression can be assessed before the cells are transplanted. Being able to genetically modify cells while they are in culture may have future potential in tailoring donor to host cells in human transplantation surgery. These experiments are being done in collaboration with Josh Dunaief from the Department of Microbiology.

CONCLUSION

Gene and cell transplantation can both lead to new forms of therapy for retinal degenerations. Both may have their place in the future in treating retinal degeneration. Cell transplantation would seem to have the advantage in those patients where the photoreceptors have all degenerated. The macula, in particular, where so much of human vision takes place would seem to be the target of choice for such research. In this case it will be cones rather than rods that should be transplanted. The success of at least three different laboratories[12-15] in achieving transplantation of rod photoreceptors implies that the transplantation of cones is also on the horizon.

ACKNOWLEDGEMENTS
We thank the The G. Harold and Leila Y. Mathers Charitable Foundation, Research to Prevent Blindness Senior Scientific Investigator Award to Dr. Peter Gouras, The Howard Hughes Medical Institute, The Bedminster Fund, Inc. and Alcon Research Institute. Anne M. Leitch for her secretarial assistance and Heinz Rosskothen for technical assistance.

REFERENCES

1. Friedmann, T., Progress toward human gene therapy, _Science_ 244, 1775, 1989.

2. Gouras, P., Flood, M.T., and Kjeldbye, H., Transplantation of human retinal cells to monkey retina. _An. Acad. Brasil. Cienc_. 56, 431, 1984.

3. Gouras, P., Lopez, R., Brittis, M., Kjeldbye, H., and Fasano, M.K., Transplantation of cultured retinal epithelium in _Retinal Signal Systems, Degenerations and Transplants_. Agardh, E., and Ehinger, B., Eds., Elsevier, Amsterdam, 1986, 271.

4. Lopez, R., Gouras, P., Brittis, M., and Kjeldbye, H., Transplantation of cultured rabbit retinal epithelium to rabbit retina using a closed eye method. _Invest. Ophthalmol. Vis. Sci_. 28, 1131, 1987.

5. Reppucci, V., Goluboff, E., Syniuta, L., Brittis, M., Sullivan, B. and Gouras, P., Retinal pigment epithelium transplantation in the RCS rat. _Invest. Ophthalmol. Vis. Sci_. 29 (suppl), 144, 1988.

6. Li, X.L. and Turner, J.E., Inherited retinal dystrophy in the RCS rat: photoreceptor cell rescue by RPE cell transplantation. _Exp. Eye Res_. 47, 911, 1988.

7. Lopez, R., Gouras, P., Kjeldbye, H., Sullivan B., Reppucci, V., Brittis, M., Goluboff, E., Transplanted retinal pigment epithelium modifies the retinal degeneration in the RCS rat. _Invest. Ophthalmol. Vis. Sci_. 30, 586, 1989.

8. Gouras, P. and Lopez, R., Editorial: Transplantation of retinal cells. _Invest. Ophthalmol. Vis. Sci_. 30, 1681, 1989.

9. Silverman, M.S. and Hughes, S.E., Photoreceptor rescue in the RCS rat without pigment epithelium transplantation. _Curr. Eye Res_. 9, 1983, 1990.

10. Faktorovich, E.G., Steinberg, R.H., Gospodarowicz, D., Yasumura, D., LaVail, M.M., Photoreceptor rescue in the RCS rat: effect of bFGF, aFGF and selected controls. _Invest. Ophthalmol. Vis. Sci_. 32(4) 595, 1990.

11. Denham, S., A cell proliferation study of the neural retina in the two-day rat. _J. Embryol. Exp. Morph_. 18, 53, 1967.

12. del Cerro, M., Notter, M.F.D., del Cerro, C., Wiegand, S.J., Grover, D.A., Lazar, E., Intraretinal transplantation for rod-cell replacement in light-damaged retina. _J. Neuro. Transpl_. 1, 1, 1989.

13.   Silverman, M.D. and Hughes, S.E., Photoreceptor transplantation in inherited and environmentally induced retinal degeneration: anatomy, histochemistry and function. in <u>Inherited and Environmentally induced retinal degenerations</u>. LaVail, M.M., Anderson, R.E. and Hollyfield J.G., Eds. Alan R. Liss, Inc. New York, 1989, 687.

14.   Gouras, P., Du, J., Gelanze, M., Lopez, R. and Kjeldbye, H., Transplantation of rods to rodless rat retina. <u>Soc. for Neurosci</u>. Abst. 15, 10, 1989.

15.   Gouras, P., Du, J., Gelanze, M., Lopez, R., Kjeldbye, H., and Krebs, W., Survival and synapse formation of transplanted rat rods. <u>J. Neurotranspl</u>. (in press).

ANALYSIS OF GENETIC HETEROGENEITY AND CLINICAL VARIATION OF TYPICAL RETINITIS PIGMENTOSA IN JAPAN

Mutsuko Hayakawa[1], Keiko Fujiki[1], Kazuyuki Kabasawa[2], Utako Tanabe[1], Atsuo Nakamura[1], Yoshihiro Hotta[1], Kazuo Kato[1], Atsushi Kanai[1] and Akira Nakajima[1]

1) Department of Ophthalmology, Juntendo University School of Medicine
   3 − 1 − 3, Hongo, Bunkyo − ku, Tokyo 113, Japan
2) Division of Information Sciences, Central Laboratory of Medical Sciences, Juntendo University School of Medicine. 3 − 1 − 3, Hongo, Bunkyo − ku, Tokyo 113, Japan

(I .) INTRODUCTION

Retinitis pigmentosa (RP) is one of the major causes of visual loss all over the world. In 1977, Matsunaga[1] analyzed the data of a Japanese RP study group consisting of 588 RP patients and reported that the prevalence of RP was estimated to be about 1 in 3400 to 1 in 8000 in Japan. The proportion of various genetic types were estimated to be 67 % autosomal recessive, 30 % autosomal dominant, and 3 % phenocopy and X − linked type.

In comparison with the distribution of genetic type of RP in England[2], USA[3] China[4] and Canada[5], more autosomal recessive and less X − linked is the characteristic of Japanese patients. During the last 33 years, the rate of first cousin marriage among the general population in Japan has decreased dramatically from about 7 % to 0.2 %[6], and the size of family has decreased rapidly. For the purpose of getting the recent information helpful for the genetic and clinical counselling, we analyzed RP patients in Juntendo University Hospital concerning the heterogeneity and phenotypic variation of typical RP. The term RP is frequently applied to various types of retinal degenerations. But in this study, we included only patients defined as typical RP whose clinical characteristics were progressive visual field loss, night blindness, midperipheral retinal bone spicule pigmentation in most, not all, narrowed retinal arterioles, and nonrecordable or abnormal ERG.

(II.) MATERIAL AND METHODS

A total of 385 patients from 379 families with typical RP seen in our clinic during the last 9 years from 1980 to 1988 were analyzed. All cases in this series were confirmed as typical RP by the clinical records. 221 were male, 164 were female, with a mean age of 40 years , and a range from 5 to 83 years old. 43 % were from Tokyo, 35 % from surrounding prefectures and the remainder from other parts of Japan. We excluded atypical RP such as sectorial form, central form and unilateral form, syndromic RP such as Usher's, Laurence-Moon-Biedle's, Refsum's syndrome and so on, related chorioretinal atrophy such as choroideremia, gyrate atrophy and retinitis punctata albescens, RP attributable to inflammation, trauma, drugs or other etiologies and the typical RP cases without family history and／or without detailed clinical record. Leber's congenital amaurosis and congenital RP with macular coloboma were also excluded to explore particular aspects of the progression of typical RP.

Patients were classified genetically on the basis of family history criteria as follows :

Autosomal recessive (AR) − one or more additional cases in sibship ; both parents and grandparents appear normal ; possible : parental consanguinity, but no affected sibs.

Autosomal dominant (AD) − direct vertical transmission through at least 2 and preferably 3 generations ; skipped generation except for the pattern of X − linked trait ; no significantly different clinical manifestations in two sexes.

X − linked (XL) − either exclusive involvement of males ; maternal grandfather, maternal uncle, maternal sister's son or brothers of proband are affected, or carrier's findings in females ; affected males transmit disorder through their daughters to grandsons ; no male to male transmission.

Simplex (Spl) − no affected relatives, no parental consanguinity.

At their initial visit, each patient had a clinical examination. To study the phenotypic variation according to the genetic type, visual acuity, visual field, age of onset, ERG, refractive error, and lens opacification were selected as parameters.

Best corrected visual acuity was divided into three groups, 0.1 or worse, 0.2~0.5, 0.6 or more, and logarithmic visual acuity was used in multivariate analysis. Visual field was recorded as the average of vertical and horizontal radii from the fovea to the isopter for the V − 4 test objects of Goldmann perimeter or 10 mm white test object of Förster perimeter, and divided into two groups, 10° or worse or more than 10° . The pattern of ERG was obtained using single flash ERG for screening in out − patient clinic and divided into two groups, recordable or nonrecordable. Refractive error was recorded as the power of glasses using to obtain the best corrected visual acuity or the power of refractometry or skiascopy. Spherical equivalence was calculated and divided into six groups, + 1.0~ + 4.75D, + 0.9~ − 0.9D, − 1.0D~ − 2.9D, − 3.0D~ − 5.9D, − 6.0D~ − 8.24D and − 8.25D~ − 15.0D. Lens opacification was divided into four groups, no opacity, mild cataract without influence on visual acuity, moderate cataract with influence on visual acuity and visible fundus, advanced cataract with invisible fundus and post extraction of cataract, by the sketch of chart and⁄or distinction of fundus photograph of each patient.

(Ⅲ.) RESULTS AND DISCUSSION

(A.) Genetic types

The proportions of genetic types were estimated to be 50 % Spl, 31 % AR, 12 % AD, 5 % XL and 2 % undermined genetic type by genetic criteria. The segregation analysis and inbreeding analysis by Fujiki[7] showed almost the same proportions. There was a higher proportion of XL and lower proportion of AR than that had been reported previously in Japan[1,8].

(B.) Clinical variation of different genetic types of RP

We investigated the phenotypic variation according to the heterogeneity of typical RP. The comparison of distribution of best corrected visual acuity group in different patient's age group, and in different duration from the onset of subjective first symptoms, among different genetic types showed the tendency that the patients of AD and Spl had less visual impairment than AR and XL (Fig.1). This result is the same as that reported by Macrae[6]. Marmor[9] reported that the progression of AD might be slightly slower than AR. The comparison of the distribution of the eye with severe field loss, 10 degrees or worse in different patient's age group and in different duration group among different genetic types showed a similar tendency as shown in visual acuity (Fig.2). A strong relationship between visual loss and visual field reported by Madreperla[10] may account for this result.

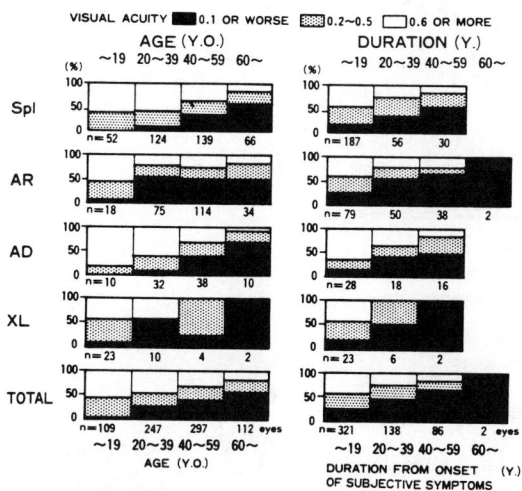

Fig. 1 DISTRIBUTION OF VISUAL ACUITY GROUP

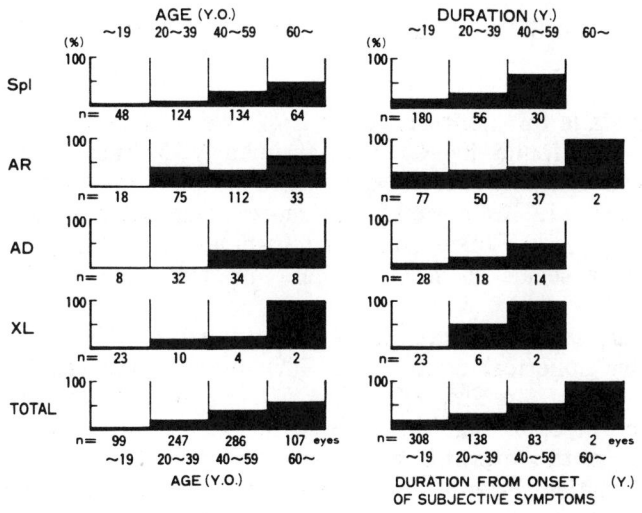

Fig. 2 DISTRIBUTION OF VISUAL FIELD ≦ 10°

The cumulative age of onset distribution of first subjective symptoms revealed that the onset of XL was significantly earlier than that of other groups (Fig.3). All patients of XL noticed the first symptoms before 20 years old and almost 60% of other groups noticed before 30 years old. There was no statistically significant difference in the age of onset among Spl, AD and AR. This result is similar to the report of Boughman and Caldwell[11] and Hu[4]. On the other hand, Berson[12] et al reported that the onset of the symptom of night blindness occured early more often in patients with AD and XL than in other affected groups. Tanino[18] reported that the age of onset of AR was significantly earlier than AD. The variabilities shown among these individual reports seem to suggest the difficulty to classify the genetic type by phenotypic criteria. Furthermore, two peaks of the age of onset were found in AR and AD in this series. This may suggest two subtypes in AR and AD.

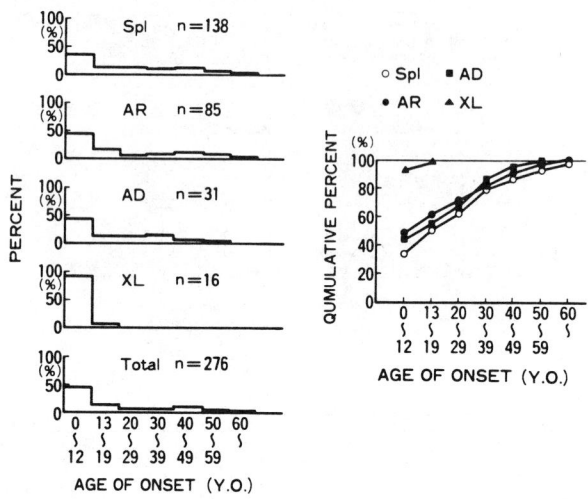

Fig. 3 AGE OF ONSET OF SUBJECTIVE SYMPTOMS OF RP PATIENTS

The percentage of nonrecordable ERG was 88.5 % of total eyes. The recordable ERG was found in AD most frequently. In the same duration group of AD comparison of early onset before 20 y.o. and late onset 20 y.o. or more showed that recordable ERG was found more frequently in late onset than in early onset. Massof and Finkelstein[14], and Fishman, et al[15] reported the subtypes of AD. This result seems to suggest there are subtypes in AD in this series.

Myopia was associated with RP frequently. 61% of RP patient had myopia of 1.0D and more spherical equivalence. The average spherical equivalences for each type were − 2.2D in Spl, − 2.2D in AR, − 1.9D in AD and − 3.7D in XL. XL had stronger myopia than the other three genetic groups. This results were similar to those in the literature[4,12,16].

40% of RP patients were found to be associated with cataract. No significant differences in the frequency of cataract were found in the different age groups among four genetic groups.

To determine the weight of influence of parameters affecting to the visual acuity, we analyzed 409 eyes using quantification theory type I (Fig.4). External criterion (Y) was visual acuity and categorized and/or concomitant variables (Xi) were visual field, ERG, cataract, age, duration from onset, age of onset, genetic type, refractive error and sex. Multiple correlation coefficient was about 0.6 and F value was 9.67, (p < 0.001). Obtained regression line was useful for estimation of visual acuity in RP. Visual acuity was influenced by in order of visual field, refractive error, duration from onset, cataract, age, age of onset and genetic type. Partial correlation coefficient showed that visual acuity had significant correlation with visual field, power of refractive error, duration from the onset and age, respectively (P < 0.01). The genetic type was found to have no statistically significant correlation with visual acuity, as reported in the Pearlman's study[17], but the direction of weight revealed there was a tendency that the visual loss of AD and Spl was milder than that of AR and XL. There was no significant correlation between visual acuity and ERG. This result seems to be attributed to the small proportion of recordable ERG in total patients.

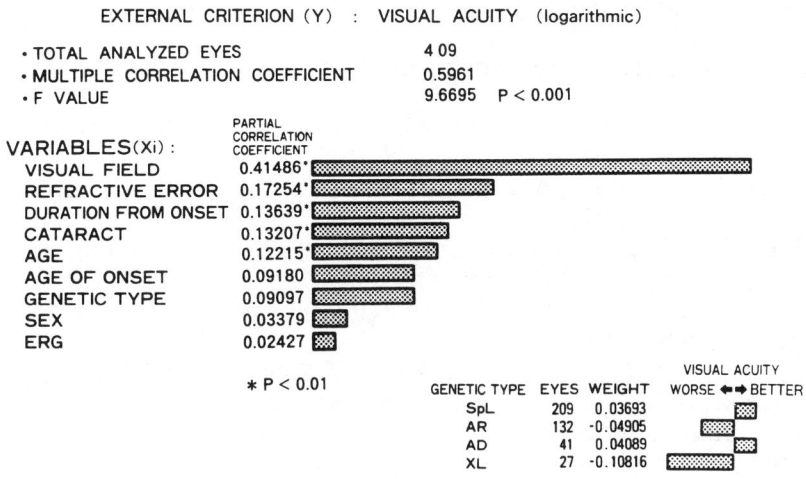

Fig. 4

MULTIVARIATE ANALYSIS IN TYPICAL RP BY QUANTIFICATION THEORY I

Genetic and clinical counselling including the perspective of natural course of an individual case is an essential part of patient care and follow − up, because effective treatment is not available in RP. These information of phenotypic variation according to the genetic type and parameters affecting visual acuity are necessary for appropriate patient care and counselling. Phenotypic variation in a given genetic type was used to catergorize subtypes of RP[16]. On the other hand, molecular biological studies revealed that there were heterogeneity in gene level in a given genetic type[18,19,20]. Study of phenotypic variation may provide the information useful for the molecular biological studies.

(IV.) SUMMARY

Distributions of various genetic types of Japanese patients were estimated to be 50 % Spl, 31 % AR, 12 % AD, and 5 % XL. The characteristics of XLRP such as earlier onset and higher myopia were found in Japanese XLRP. Recordable ERG was found in AD most frequently, especially in late onset AD. There was no significant difference of age of onset among Spl, AD and AR. Multivariate analysis by quantification theory I showed that visual acuity was influenced by in order of visual field, power of refractive error, duration from onset, cataract, age, and genetic type. There were significant correlation between visual acuity and visual field, power of refractive error, duration from onset, cataract and age respectively. There was the tendency that visual loss of AD and Spl was milder than AR and XL.

ACKNOWLEDGMENT

This work was supported by a grant for chorioretinal degeneration from the Japanese Ministry of Health and Welfare.

REFERENCE

1. Matsunaga, N., Genetic study on retinitis pigmentosa, <u>Annual Report to Retinitis Pigmentosa Study Group, Ministry of Health and Welfare, Government of Japan</u>, 119, 1977.
2. Jay, M., On the heredity of retinitis pigmentosa, <u>Br. J. Ophthalmol.</u>, 66, 405 1982.
3. Boughman, J.A., Fishman G.A., A genetic analysis of retinitis pigmentosa, <u>Br. J. Ophthalmol.</u>, 67, 449, 1983.
4. Hu, D.N., Genetic aspects of retinitis pigmentosa in China, <u>Am. J. Med. Genet.</u>, 12, 51, 1982.
5. Macrae, W.G., Retinitis pigmentosa in Ontario − A survey, Birth Defects, Original article series, 18, 175, 1982.
6. Imaizumi, Y., A recent survey of consanguineous marriage in Japan, <u>Clin. Genet.</u>, 30, 230, 1986.
7. Fujiki, K., Hayakawa M., Hotta, Y., Tanabe, U., Kanai, A. and Nakajima A., Primary retinitis pigmentosa in Japan, presented at poster session, International Ophthalmology Congress, Singapore, March 19 − 23, 1990.
8. Ohba, N. and Tanino, T., Genetic heterogeneity of pigmentary retinal dystrophy : analysis of the mode of inheritance in 104 pedigrees, <u>Jpn. J. Ophthalmol.</u> 79, 1807, 1975.
9. Marmer, M.F., Visual loss in retinitis pigmentosa., <u>Amer. J. Ophthalmol.</u>, 89, 692, 1980.
10. Madreperla, S.A., Visual acuity loss in retinitis pigmentosa, Relationship to visual field loss, <u>Arch. Ophthalmol.</u> 108, 358, 1990.
11. Boughman, J.A. and Caldwell, R.J., Assessment of clinical variables and counselling needs in patients with retinitis pigmentosa, <u>Amer. J. Med. Genet.</u>, 12, 185, 1982.
12. Berson, E. L., Rosner, B., Simonoff, E., Risk factors for genetic typing and detection in retinitis pigmentosa, <u>Am. J. Ophthalmol.</u> 89, 763, 1980.
13. Tanino, T., Ohba, N., Studies on pigmentary retinal dystrophy, I. Age of onset of subjective symptom and the mode of inheritance, <u>Jap. J. Ophthalmol.</u>, 20, 474, 1976.
14. Massof, R.W. and Finkelstein, D., Two forms of autosomal dominant primary retinitis pigmentosa. <u>Doc. Ophthalmol.</u>, 51, 289, 1981.
15. Fishman, G.A., Alexander, K.R., and Anderson, R.J., Autosomal dominant retinitis pigmentosa, A method of classification, <u>Arch. Ophthalmol.</u>, 130, 366, 1985.
16. Sieving, P.A., and Fishman, G.A., Refractive errors of retinitis pigmentosa patients, <u>Br. J. Ophthalmol.</u>, 62, 163, 1978.
17. Pearlman, J.T., Mathematical models of retinitis pigmentosa, Study of the rate of progressive in different genetic forms, <u>Trans. Am. Ophthalmol. Soc.</u>, 77, 643, 1979.
18. McWilliam, P., Farrar, G.J., Kenna, P., Bradley, D.G., Humphries, M.M., Sharp, E.M., McConnell, D.J., Lawler, M., Sheils, D., Ryan, C., Stevens, K., Daiger, S. P. and Humphries, P., Autosomal dominant retinitis pigmentosa ; Localization of an ADRP gene to the long arm of chromosom 3, <u>Genomics</u> 5, 619, 1989.
19. Inglehearn, C.F., Jay, M., Lester, D.H., Bashir, R., Jay, B., Bird, A.C., Wright, A.F., Evans, H.J., Papiha, S. S. and Bhattacharya, S.S., No evidence for linkage

between late onset autosomal dominant retinitis pigmentosa and chromosome 3 locus D3S47 (C17) : Evidence for Genetic Heterogeneity, <u>Genomics,</u> 6, 168, 1990.

20. Dryja, T.P., McGee, T.L., Reichel, E., Hahn, L.B., Cowley G.S., Yandell W., Sandberg, M.A. and Berson, E.L., A point mutation of the rhodopsin gene in one form of retinitis pigmentosa, <u>Nature,</u> 343, 364, 1990.

LINKAGE ANALYSIS IN AUTOSOMAL DOMINANT RETINITIS PIGMENTOSA

J.KAPLAN*, G.GUASCONI*, JL. DUFIER***, A. AWAD-MICHEL***, A. DAVID**, A. MUNNICH*, and J. FREZAL*

* INSERM U.12 Unité de Recherches sur les Handicaps génétiques de l'enfant Hôpital des Enfants Malades - PARIS, ** Service de Pédiatrie - CHU Nantes, *** Consultation d'Ophtalmologie - Hôpital Laënnec - PARIS

INTRODUCTION

Autosomal dominant forms of retinitis pigmentosa (RP) are progressive retinal degenerations considered as rod-cone dystrophies. Rods are found on the whole retina except the macula. They are responsible for night vision and peripheral visual field. The electroretinographic expression of rod impairment is an alteration or absence of the so-called "scotopic response". During the course of RP, night blindness occurs with progressive narrowing of the visual field. Fundus examination shows the abnormal presence of dark pigments (bone spicule pigmentation) from which the name of the condition is derived. These lesions correspond to the primary impairment of rods, followed by depigmentation of the pigmented epithelium with displacement of small clumps of pigment towards the deepest layers of the retina.[1] Cones are largely found in macula and are responsible for visual acuity, colour discrimination and tolerance of bright light. The electroretinographic expression of cone impairment is an alteration of the so-called "photopic response". Two clinical subtypes of autosomal dominant RP (ADRP) could be distinguished according to the delay in macular involvement. In the severe form, macular involvement occured within 10 years, while in the mild form, macular involvement occured after 20 years of evolution.[2] The clinical heterogeneity observed in ADRP may be either paralleled by genetic heterogeneity or due to allelic mutations at the same locus.

In a large Irish family the gene for ADRP I has been recently assigned to the long arm of chromosome 3, closely linked to D3S47 (probe C17, Mac William, 1989).[3] More recently, Dryja, 1990,[4] has demonstrated the first point mutation of RP in the rhodopsin gene as a $C \rightarrow A$ transversion in codon 23 corresponding to a proline→histidine substitution.

In our study the C17 probe was used first for testing a possible linkage with ADRP type II, and no linkage was found with this particular probe, suggesting a genetic heterogeneity of autosomal dominant RP.

On the other hand C17 probe was used in one family of ADRP type I and we found a probable linkage suggesting the location of the gene in this family on chromosome 3q.

MATERIAL AND METHODS

Two families of ADRP II were ascertained through the Association Française Retinitis Pigmentosa (AFRP). For each of them, the medical data were analysed, a detailed history was obtained by interview of several affected individuals, and a pedigree was established. Minimal criteria for the diagnosis of RP was night blindness as mode of onset at a mean-age of 12 years, a progressive narrowing of the visual field and abnormal presence of dark pigments with attenuation of retina vessels at the fundus examination. In addition most of affected subjects exhibited a severely reduced electroretinogram (ERG) while a reasonably good central vision was conserved for several decades. These two families include 17 live affected subjects, 12 live healthy sibs and 8 husbands and wifes (figure 1).

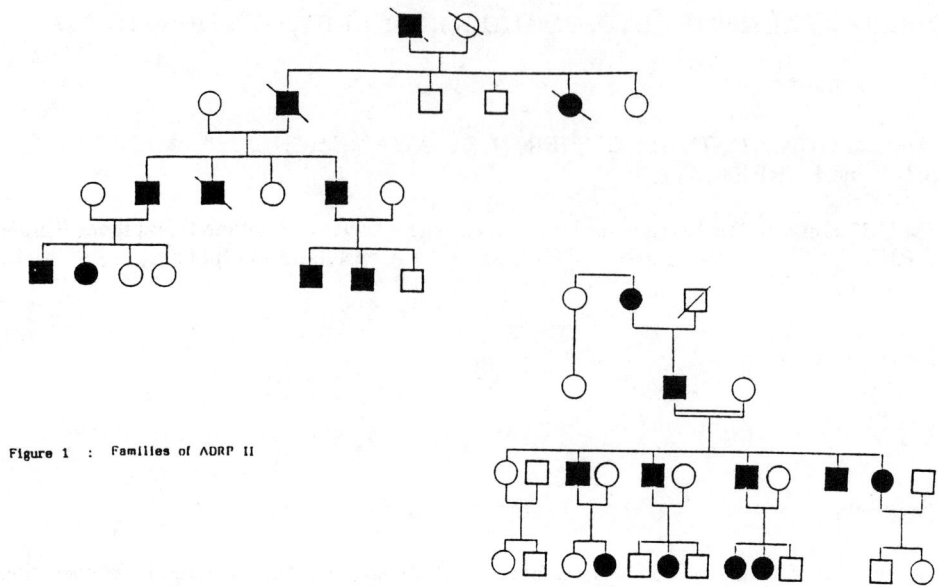

Figure 1 : Families of ADRP II

On the other hand one family of ADRP I was studied, including 5 live affected individuals, 2 healthy sibs and 4 non examined infants (figure 2). All affected members displayed an early night blindness as mode of onset at a mean-age of 4 years, a fast narrowing of visual field and a reduced central vision before 30 years. All of them exhibited an extinguished ERG at an early stage. Blood samples were obtained from 51 individuals belonging to these 3 families.

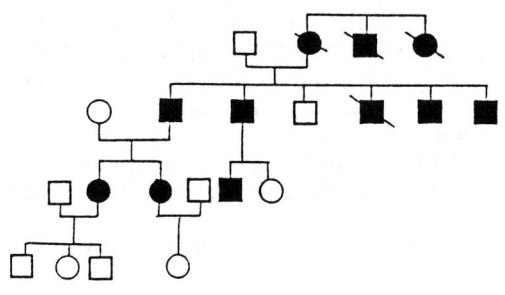

Figure 2 : Family of ADRP I

For restriction fragment length polymorphism (RFLP) analysis, DNA was extracted from lymphocyte pellets by cell lysis, proteinase K digestion, phenol/chloroform extraction, ethanol precipitation and tris-EDTA resuspension. DNA (5 µg) was cleaved with the restriction enzyme Msp I under appropriate buffer and temperature conditions according to the manufacturer's recommandations. The fragments vere separated by horizontal gel electrophoresis in Tris-acetate EDTA buffer and transfered onto a nylon membrane (Zetabind, Flo Cuno) using Southern's technique. Probes vere radiolabeled by nick-translation to a high specific activity with $32p$ -dCTP (Amersham). After hybridization, the filters were washed and exposed to KODAK X/OMAT films with intensifying screens. Linkage analysis was carried out using the LINKAGE program version 4.8[5] on a IBM PC AT.

RESULTS

Table 1 shows the results of two-point linkage calculation between ADRP II and the C17 polymorphism. Lod-scores were negative at θ = 0.001 (Z = -9.46) and still negative values vere found to all values of θ. It is clear that the polymorphism identified by probe C17 is not linked in our families of ADRP II.

Table 1 : LOD SCORES BETWEEN ADRPII and C 17

	0	0.001	0.01	0.05	0.1	0.2	0.3
Fam 1	- ∞	- 4.50	- 2.51	- 1.16	- 0.63	- 0.18	- 0.005
Fam 2	- ∞	- 4.96	- 2.96	- 1.57	- 0.99	- 0.44	- 0.17
Fam 1+2	- ∞	- 9.46	- 5.47	- 2.73	- 1.62	- 0.62	- 0.18

Table 2 shows the results of two-point linkage calculation between our family of ADRP I and the C17 polymorphism. A peak lod score of Z = 1.50 was obtained at θ = 0.

Owing to the small number of individuals, this lod score does not allow to firmly establish a linkage between the disease gene and probe C17 in this family. However in this particular family, a further argument in favour of linkage may be found in the observation of a modification in the restriction site with this probe : all affected members do not display the usual alleles of the polymorphism since they have lost one of them. In contrast, they exhibited abnormal bands. The sum in kb of these abnormal bands is equal to the missed usual band. (figure 3).

Table 2 : Lod-scores between
one family of ADRP I and C 17

	0	0.05	0.1	0.2	$\hat{z}$	$\hat{\theta}$
ADRPI - C 17	1.50	1.34	1.18	0.83	1.50	0

Figure 3 :   RPDA I - D3S47 (CRI-C17)

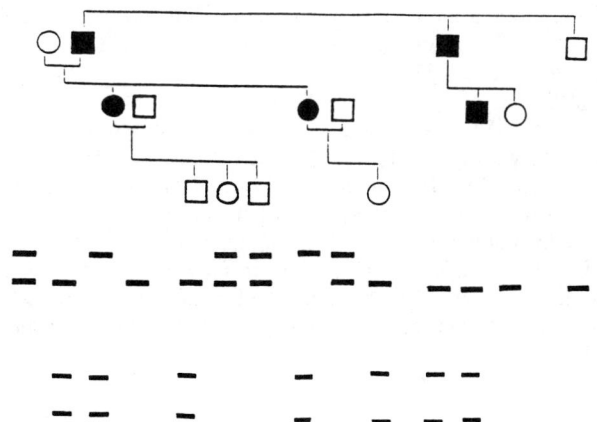

DISCUSSION

Autosomal dominant RP has been previously clinically subclassified into two groups on the basis of psychophysical testing and age of onset.[6,7,8] ADRP type I is characterized by a diffuse loss of rod sensitivity, later loss of cone sensitivity, and early onset in childhood.By contrast, ADRP type II is characterized by a regional loss of both rod and cone sensitivity with later onset of night-blindness in adulthood.

In a large series of 93 independant families with RP,[1] we have recognized two clinical forms of ADRP according to their clinical course. The difference does not lie on the age or type of onset symptom (which is consistently night-blindness il all patients) but rather on the clinical course of the disease. In fact, the course of type I is markedly accelerated for both concentric loss of the visual field and macular involvement. Indeed, macular involvement in type I accurs within 10 years while in type II, it always occurs after 20 years of evolution. This difference is highly significant and accounts for severity of type I.[2]

These findings, associated to the exclusion data found in our two families of ADRP II, unambiguously reject the linkage of this type of moderate-late onset ADRP to the C17 locus and are in agreement with the study of Inglehearn.[9]

By contrast our peak lod score of 1.50 found at $\theta = 0$ in our family of ADRP I (5 certainly affected members, 2 healthy sibs and 4 ambiguous infants) suggests a probable linkage of this more severe type of ADRP to the C17 locus.

In conclusion in this study we demonstrate that ADRP type I and type II are not located at the same locus on chromosome 3, thus excluding allelic mutations as the cause of the two phenotypes. The question of whether a genetic heterogeneity also exists in type I, remains open to debate, especially since, according to Dryja, 1990, quite different point mutations seem have been found in C17 - linked ADRP I.

We are thankful to Cécile Glaunec and Marie-Sophie Baule for their help in preparing this manuscript. The present study was supported by the Association Française Retinitis Pigmentosa.

REFERENCES

1. Pagon, R.A., Retinitis pigmentosa, Surv. Ophtalmol., 33, 137, 1988.
2. Kaplan, J., Bonneau, D., Frézal, J., Munnich, A., Dufier, J.L., Clinical and genetic heterogeneity in retinitis pigmentosa, Hum. Genet, 1990 (in press)
3. Mc William, P., Farrar, G.J., Kenna, P., Bradley, D.G., Humphries, M.M., Sharp, E.M., Mc Connell, D.J., Lawler, M., Sheils, D., Ryan, C., Stevens, K., Daiger, S.P., Humphries, P., Autosomal dominant retinitis pigmentosa (ADRP) : localization of an ADRP gene to the long arm of chromosome 3, Genomics, 5, 619, 1989.
4. Dryja, T.P., Mc Gee, T.L., Reichel, E., Hahn, L.B., Cowley, G.S., Yandell, D.W., Sandberg, M.A., Berson, E.L., A point mutation of the rhodopsin gene in one form of retinitis pigmentosa, Nature, 343, 364, 1990.
5. Lathrop, G.M., Lalouel, J.M., Easy calculation of lod-scores and genetic risks on small computers, Am. J. Hum. Genet., 36, 460, 1984.
6. Massof, R.W., Finkelstein, D., Two forms of autosomal dominant primary retinitis pigmentosa, Doc. Ophtalmol., 51, 289, 1981.
7. Farber, M.D., Fishman, G.A., Weiss, R.A., Autosomal dominant inherited retinitis pigmentosa : visual acuity loss by subtype, Arch. Ophtalmol., 103, 524, 1985.
8. Lyness, A.L., Ernest, W., Quinlan, M.P., Clover, G.M., Arden, G.B., Carter, R.M., Bird, A.C., Parker, J.A., A clinical, psychophysical, and electroretinographic survey of patients with autosomal dominant retinitis pigmentosa, Br. J. Ophtalmol., 69, 326, 1985.
9. Inglehearn,C.F., Jay, M., Lester, D.H., Bashir, R., Jay, B., Bird, A.C., Wright, A.F., Evans, H.J., Papiha, S.S., Bhattacharya, S.S., No evidence for linkage between late onset autosomal dominant retinitis pigmentosa and chromosome 3 locus D3S47 (C17) : evidence for genetic heterogeneity, Genomics, 6,168, 1990.

LINKAGE ANALYSIS IN USHER SYNDROME TYPE I

J. KAPLAN*, G. GUASCONI*, D. BONNEAU**, J. MELKI*, ML BRIARD*, JL DUFIER***, A. MUNNICH*, and J. FREZAL*

* INSERM U.12 Unité de Recherches sur les Handicaps génétiques de l'enfant Hôpital des Enfants Malades - PARIS, ** Service de Pédiatrie - CHU Poitiers, *** Consultation d'Ophtalmologie - Hôpital Laënnec - PARIS

INTRODUCTION

Usher syndrome (US) is an autosomal recessive disease characterized by a congenital sensorineural hearing impairment, progressive visual loss secondary to retinitis pigmentosa, and sometimes involvement of the vestibular system. It is considered as the most frequent cause of deaf-blindness in adults and affects 5 to 10 % of deaf children. It involves about 14 % of patients with a retinal degenerative disorder.[1]

Affected individuals have a sensorineural hearing loss, present at birth, and later develop a typical retinitis pigmentosa which usually occurs ten years after the discovery of deafness. Two clinical forms have been recognized namely a) congenital and severe (type I) and b) late and moderate (type II). (Table 1).[2,3]

Recently, Kimberling et al.[4] reported on the mapping of the type II Usher syndrome gene to the long arm of chromosome 1, by linkage with an anonymous DNA marker D1S81 (probe THH 33). A maximum lod-score of $\hat{Z} = 6.04$ was obtained at $\hat{\theta} = 0$.

Simultanously, Lewis et al.[5] tested this probe in 22 families of US type II and found the same linkage with a maximum lod-score of $\hat{Z} = 6.5$ at $\hat{\theta} = 0.09$.

First, in the present study, the THH 33 probe was used for testing a possible linkage with US type I, and no linkage was found with this particular probe, suggesting a genetic heterogeneity of Usher disease[6] as previously mentioned by Kimberling and Lewis.

Second, in order to contribute to the localization of US type I locus, we have analysed our pedigrees using polymorphic DNA markers located on the long arm of chromosome 14 and we have looked for a possible linkage with this chromosome.

Table 1 : CLINICAL SUBTYPES of USHER DISEASE

Clinical feature	Type I	Type II
Hearing-loss	congenital, profound	congenital, moderate
Language	no	yes
Vestibular function	absent or abnormal	normal
Onset of retinitis pigmentosa	1st decade or beginning of the 2nd	end of 2nd decade or beginning of the 3rd
Ataxia	occasional	absent
Mental retardation	occasional	absent
Psychosis	occasional	absent

MATERIAL and METHODS

Six families of US were ascertained through the Poitiers school for Deaf and Blind Children (figure 1). For each of them, the medical data were analysed, a detailed history was obtained by interviewing the parents, and a pedigree was established. Minimal criteria for the diagnosis of US type I were a) deafness and dumbness discovered in the first eighteen months of life, requiring reeducation of language, and b) evidence of retinitis pigmentosa at ophthalmological investigation. Because of the severity of the disease the distinction between affected and non-affected members was clearcut and unambiguous. This study includes 29 individuals, 8 of whom are affected children (figure 1).

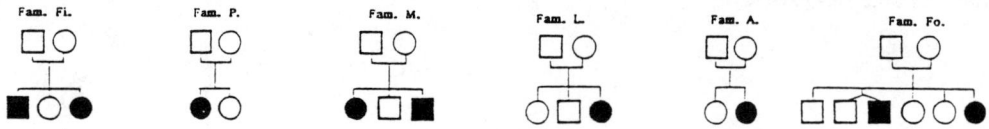

Figure 1 : Pedigrees of Usher type I
analysed in this study

A 20 ml EDTA-blood sample was collected from each of the 29 individuals. DNAs were prepared from lymphocyte pellets by SDS lysis, proteinase K digestion, phenol/chloroform extraction, ethanol precipitation, and tris EDTA resuspension. DNA (5 μg) was cleaved with the restriction enzymes Rsa I, Msp I and Bam HI under appropriate buffer and temperature conditions according to the manufacterer's recommandations. DNA fragments were separated by horizontal gel electrophoresis in TEA buffer, stained with ethidium bromide for visual inspection and denatured in situ with 0.25 N HCl. The denatured DNA fragments were transfered on to a nylon membrane (Zetabind, Flo Cuno) using Southern's technique. The DNA probe was labeled with 32P dCTP by nick-translation and purified on a Sephadex G-50 column to remove unincorporated nucleotides. The labeled plasmid was then competitively hybridized to sheared total human DNA to reduce lane background caused by common repeats in the probe[7]. The mix was then added to 25 ml of the hybridization solution. Membranes were hybridized in polythene bags overnight at 65°C. They were washed twice at room temperature in 2 x SSEP and 0.1 % SDS, then washed at 65°C in 1 x SSEP and 0.1 % SDS. Autoradiographs were obtained by exposure to Kodak X/OMAT films for 1-4 days at -80°C.

The probes and some of their relevant characteristics are listed in table 2. Linkage analysis was performed using the linkage program version 4.8[8] on an IBM PC AT.

Table 2 : polymorphic DNA markers used

Locus	probe	location	enzyme	polymorphism
D1 S81	THH 33	1q	Rsa I	VNTR with > 10 alleles heterozygosity = 0.85
D14 S23	KKA 39	14q 32.32 – q 32.33	Msp I	VNTR with > 10 alleles heterozygosity = 0.83
D14 S13	MLJ 14	14q 32	Rsa I	VNTR with > 20 alleles heterozygosity = 0.95
TCRD	DV2SPO.5	14q 11.2	Bam III	3 alleles PIC = 0.46

RESULTS

Table 3 shows the results of two-point linkage calculation between the US type I gene and the pTHH 33 polymorphism. Lod-scores were negative at $\theta = 0.001$ ($Z = -6.80$) and still negative values were found up to a recombination fraction of 0.40. It is clear that the polymorphism identified by probe pTHH 33 is not linked to the US type I gene in our families.

Table 4 shows the results of two-point linkage analysis between the US type 1 locus and three polymorphic DNA markers on chromosome 14 q. Nowadays the lod-scores found in this study are not significant neither for a linkage nor an exclusion of linkage, since the peak lod score does not reach the accepted log likelihood of 3 for linkage or by contrast of -2 for exclusion.

Table 3 :   LOD-SCORES BETWEEN

pTHH 33 RFLP AND US TYPE I FAMILIES

0	0.001	0.01	0.05	0.1	0.2	0.3	0.4
$-\infty$	-6.80	-3.80	-1.74	-0.94	-0.31	-0.09	-0.016

Table 4   :   LINKAGE USHER I - CHROM 14 q

	0	0.05	0.1	0.2	$\hat{Z}$	$\hat{\theta}$
USHI-KKA39	$-\infty$	-0.22	0.13	0.23	0.24	0.18
USHI-MLJ14	$-\infty$	-0.72	0.73	0.49	0.75	0.07
USHI- DV2SPO.5	0.93	0.81	0.69	0.46	0.93	0

DISCUSSION

Some investigators believe that US is subdivided in at least four types with types I to III being autosomal recessive and based on phenotypic variations[9,10,11], while type IV differs by its mode of inheritance. In this classification, type III is characterized by progressive and variable hearing loss with retinitis pigmentosa also being variable in its age of occurrence. Type IV is clinically similar to type II but is X-linked.[12] Unfortunately, only one publication is available regarding this mode of inheritance and no other pedigrees have been reported thus far. If this form does exist, it could be difficult to distinguish it from the autosomal recessive forms, in sibships with males only being affected. US type I, however, cannot be misdiagnosed because it is the only form with profound congenital deafness and early retinitis pigmentosa.

For these reasons, the exclusion data presented here, along with the independant data from Kimberling et al.[4] and Lewis et al.[5], unambiguously reject the linkage of type I US to the THH 33 locus. Taken together, these different results support the view that the clinical heterogeneity of US is accounted for by an obvious genetic heterogeneity.

On account of this genetic heterogeneity, the task of searching for linkage in Usher type I must continue. We present here the first results of a pairwise linkage study between US I and three mapped markers on chromosome 14. This study is still in progress and we intend to look for linkage with other probes on chromosome 14 q. Effectively, our preliminary data are not able to suggest or to exclude a possible location of the US I gene on this chromosome.

On the other hand we have increased the number of our families affected by Usher type I, in order to reduce the problem of informativity with the polymorphic probes studied here. Indeed, it is interesting to note that we have found a peak lod-score of $Z = 0.93$ at $\theta = 0$ between TCRD (probe DV2SPO.5) and only two families of Usher type I (Fam L. and Fam Fo, figure 1), the four other families beeing not informative with this probe.

Finally our pairwise analysis will be completed by multipoint analysis assuming, first, equal male and female recombination rates, with distances fixed from the sex-averaged genetic map of Donis-Keller et al.[13], and second, assuming sex-specific differences in recombination frequency. This multipoint analysis will give us a better support either for linkage or for exclusion between US type I locus and chromosome 14 q.

In conclusion, this study demonstrates that US type I and US type II genes are not located at the same locus on chromosome 1, thus excluding allelic mutations as the cause of the two phenotypes. This genetic heterogeneity within US is therefore in striking contrast with other clinically related genetic diseases, such as Duchenne and Becker muscular dystrophies[14] and spinal muscular atrophies types II and III[15] where allelism has been clearly demonstrated.

In addition we supply the first preliminary data for tentative of linkage of Usher type I. This work for linkage must be carried on, and we should appreciate cooperation in order to extend our sample and definitely settle the point.

We are grateful to Dr MP Lefranc, and to Drs Y. Nakamura and R. White for providing the probes used in this study.

We are also thankful to the physicians in charge of deaf and blind children in the Institution of Poitiers, and to Cécile Glaunec and Marie-Sophie Baule for their help in preparing this manuscript. the present study was supported by the Association Française Retinitis Pigmentosa.

REFERENCES

1. Kaplan, J., Bonneau, D., Frézal, J., Munnich, A., Dufier, JL., Clinical and genetic heterogeneity in retinitis pigmentosa, Hum. Genet., 1990 (in press).
2. Merin, S., Abraham, F.A., Auerbach, E., Usher's and Hallgren's syndromes, Acta. Genet. Med. Gemell, 23, 49, 1974.
3. Fishmann, G.A., Kummar, A., Joseph, M.E., Torak, N., Anderson, R.J., Usher's syndrome ophtalmic and neuro-otologic findings suggesting genetic heterogeneity, Arch. Ophtalmol., 101, 1367, 1983.
4. Kimberling, W.J., Weston, M.D., Moller, C., Davenport, S.L.H., Shugart, Y.Y., Priluck, I.A., Martini, A., Milani, M., Smith, R.J., Localization of Usher syndrome type II to chromosome 1q, Genomics, 7, 245, 1990.
5. Lewis, R.A., Otterud, B., Stauffer, D., Lalouel, J.M., Leppert, M., Mapping recessive opthalmic diseases : linkage of the locus for Usher syndrome type II to a DNA marker on chromosome 1q, Genomics, 7, 250, 1990.
6. Kaplan, J., Guasconi, G., Bonneau, D., Melki, J., Briard, M.L., Munnich, A., Dufier, J.L., and Frézal, J., Usher syndrome type I is not linked to D1S81 (pTHH 33) : evidence for genetic heterogeneity, Ann. Genet., 33, 2, 1990.
7. Sealey, P.G., Whittaker, P.A., Southern, E.M., Removal of repeat sequences from hybridisation probes, Nucleic Acids Res., 13, 1905, 1985.
8. Lathrop, G.M., Lalouel, J.M., Easy calculation of lod-scores and genetic risks on small computers, Am. J. Hum. Genet., 36, 460, 1984.
9. Nuutila, A., Dystropia retinae pigmentosa-dysacussis syndrome (DRD) : a study of the Usher or Hallgren syndrome, J. Genet. Hum., 118, 57, 1970.
10. Nance, W.E., Genetic aspects of Usher's syndrome in symposium of Usher's syndrome, Gallaudet College, Washington DC 1973.
11. Gorlin, R.J., Tilsnert, T.J., Feinstein, S., Duvall, A.J., Usher's syndrome type III, Arch. Otolaryngol., 105, 353, 1979.

12. Davenport, S.L.H., O'Naullain, S., Omenn, G.S., Wilkus, R.J., Usher syndrome in four hard-of-hearing siblings, Pediatrics, 62, 578, 1978.

13. Donis-Keller, H., Green, P., Helms, C., Cartinhour, S., Weiffenbach, B., Stephens, K., Keith, T.P., Bowden, D.W., Smith, D.R., Lander, E.S., Botstein, D., Akots, G., Rediker, K.S., Gravus, T., Brown, V.A., Rising, M.B., Parker, C., Powers, J.A., Watt, D.E., Kauffman, E.R., Bricker, A., Phipps, P., Muller-Kahle, H., Fulton, T.R., NG, S., Schumm, J.W., Braman, J.C., Knowlton, R.G., Barker, D.F., Crooks, S.M., Lincoln, S.E., Daly, M.J., and Abrahamson, J., A genetic linkage map of the human genome, Cell, 51, 319, 1987.

14. Fadda, S., Mochi, M., Roncuzzi, L., Sangiorgi, S., Sbarra, D., Zatz, M., Romeo, G., Definitive localization of Becker muscular dystrophy in Xp by linkage to a cluster of DNA polymorphisms (DXS43 and DXS9), Hum. Genet., 71, 33, 1985.

15. Melki, J., Abderhak, S., Sheth, P., Bachelot, M.F., Burlet, P., Marcadet, A., Aicardi, J., Barois, A., Carriere, J.P., Fardeau, M., Fontan, D., Ponsot, G., Billette, T., Angelini, C., Barbosa, C., Ferriere, G., Lanzi, G., Ottolini, A., Babron, M.C., Cohen, D., Hanauer, A., Clerget-Darpoux, F., Lathrop, M., Munnich, A., Frézal, J., Gene for chronic proximal spinal muscular atrophies maps to chromosome 5q, Nature, 344, 767, 1990.

CHARACTERISATION OF IRISH AUTOSOMAL DOMINANT RETINITIS PIGMENTOSA KINDREDS SHOWING GENETIC HETEROGENEITY

PAUL F. KENNA F. R. C. S. I.

Department of Genetics, Trinity College Dublin,Ireland and Research Department, Royal Victoria Eye and Ear Hospital, Dublin

Introduction

Autosomal dominant kindreds have been ascertained and characterized at the Research Department of the Royal Victoria Eye and Ear Hospital, Dublin. The two largest of these (Fig. 1 and 2) have been used for linkage analysis at the Department of Genetics at Trinity College, Dublin.[1, 2, 3] These two kindreds differ in clinical characteristics and have demonstrated genetic heterogeneity with Chromosome 3q markers, TCD M showing tight linkage and TCD G exclusion.[1, 4]

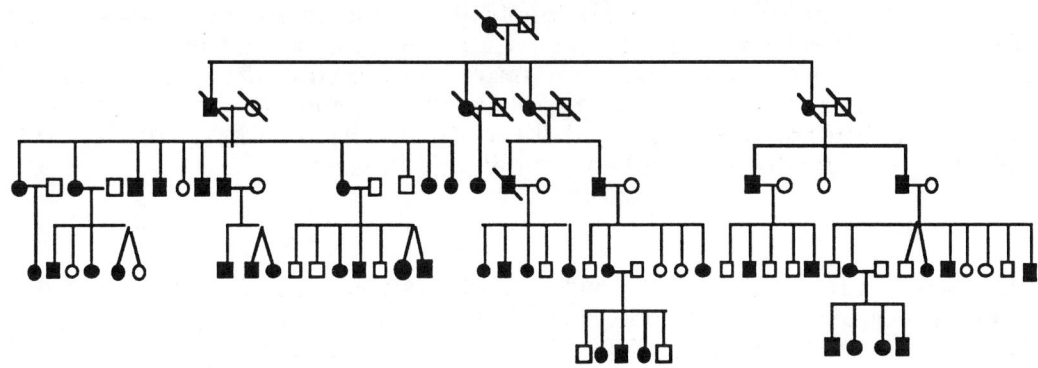

Figure 1 TCD M

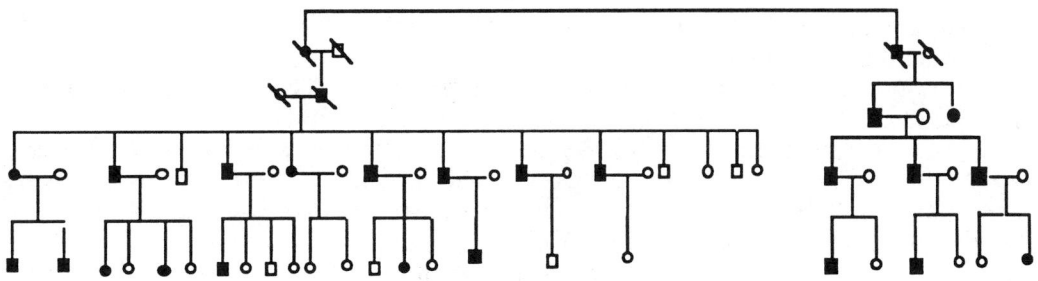

Figure 2 TCD G

Materials and Methods

Ophthalmological examination of individuals from both pedigrees included corrected visual acuity, colour vision assessment, Goldmann perimetry, slit-lamp biomicroscopy, dark adaptometry, direct and indirect fundoscopy, and fundus photography. Electroretinography (ERG) was performed using the protocol described by Arden et al.[5] Briefly, the pupils were dilated with Tropicamide and the subject was dark adapted for 20 minutes. Gold foil corneal electrodes were inserted under dim red illumination. Rod isolated responses were elicited by low intensity blue flashes. Combined rod and cone responses were elicited by maximal intensity white flashes. Cone responses were assessed by 30Hz white flickers. Responses were computer averaged.

Certain affected individuals in both pedigrees had monocular two colour dark adaptometry performed using a protocol described by Sondheimer et al.[6] Red (Kodak gel filter 80A) and blue (Kodak gel filter 21) test targets in a Goldmann - Weekers dark adaptometer were used. A retinal locus 15° above fixation was tested for the first 30 minutes. Loci at 30° and 45° above fixation, 15°, 30° and 45° below fixation and 15° from fixation in the 45°-225° and 135°-315° meridians were assessed after 30 minutes. The intensity at which the subject first noted the stimulus was determined, then the intensity at which the subject ceased to see the target. These intensities were measured twice and the true absolute threshold was taken as the average of the two intensities for each testing. At each testing the rod mediated (blue) threshold was determined first, then the cone mediated (red) threshold was measured.

Results

The two kindreds differed most notably in the age of onset of night blindness and in their two colour dark adaptometry profiles.

All affected individuals in TCD M, without exception, reported night blindness from earliest childhood. Mothers volunteered that they could predict which of their offspring was affected by the manner in which they coped with low light situations once they had become mobile. Despite this very early onset of night blindness, affected individuals retain good central vision until the 5th or 6th decades. None demonstrates nystagmus.

In contrast, affected individuals in the pedigree TCD G did not report difficulties with night vision until their late 20s or early 30s.

ERG recordings from individuals as young as 6 years in TCD M show extinguished rod and cone responses (Fig. 3 A). Tracings from young affecteds in TCD G by contrast, demonstrate recordable, albeit reduced amplitude, rod responses (Fig. 3B).

The pattern of two colour dark adaptometry shows marked differences between the two kindreds. Young affected individuals (2nd decade) in TCD M show elevation of both rod and cone thresholds, with greater elevation of the rod threshold. This pattern is observed in all retinal loci tested (Fig. 5). TCD G affecteds demonstrate a distinctly different pattern

tested (Fig. 5). TCD G affecteds demonstrate a distinctly different pattern with elevation of both rod and cone thresholds but in a patchy manner. Some retinal loci show normal or near normal thresholds (Fig. 6). The profile of an unaffected individual is shown in Fig. 4.

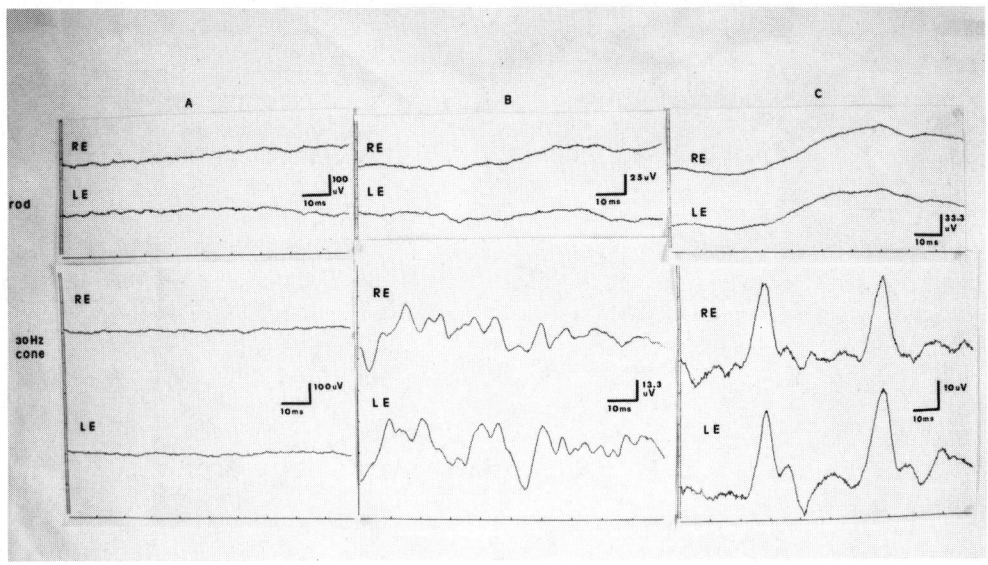

Figure 3 A) TCD M affected B) TCD G affected C) Normal

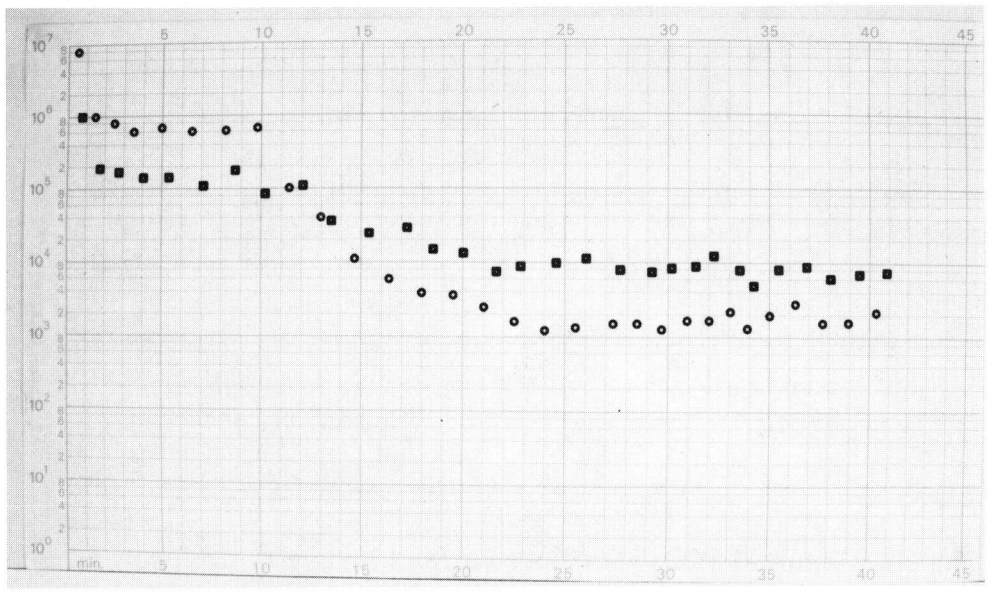

Figure 4 Normal 2 colour dark adaptometry profile
o = Rod (blue) threshold
■ = Cone (red) threshold

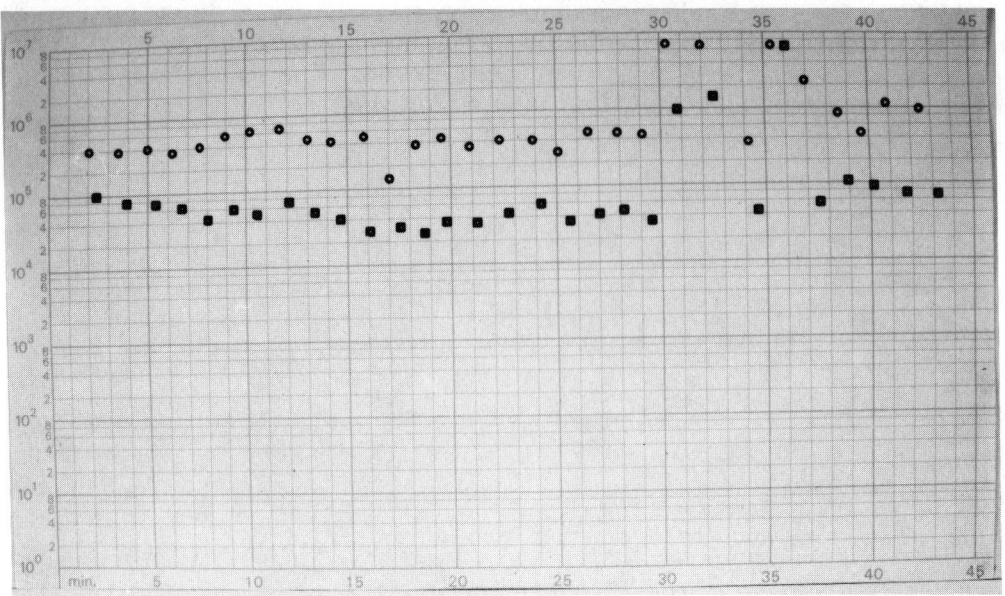

Figure 5 TCD M 2 colour dark adaptometry profile

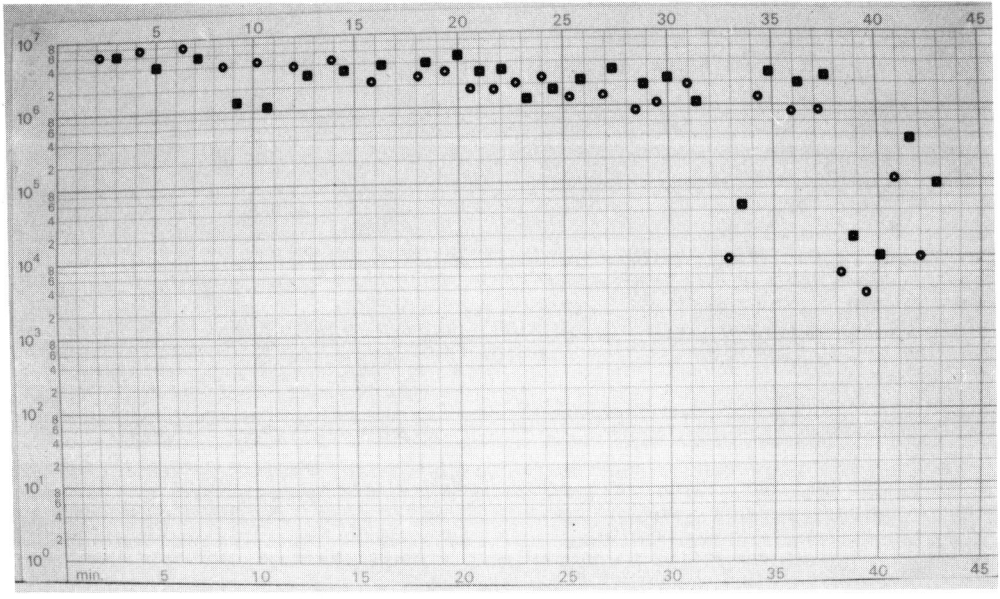

Figure 6 TCD G 2 colour dark adaptometry profile

Discussion

Autosomal Dominant Retinitis Pigmentosa (ADRP) has been thought to be a clinically heterogeneous condition for some time. Various sub - divisions have been suggested in the past based on penetrance,[7] ERG criteria[8,9] or psychophysical profiles.[10,11]

Massof and Finkelstein[10] divided 25 ADRP patients into two sub - groups based on their relative rod and cone sensitivities as determined by two colour dark adapted static perimetry. Type 1 patients had an early, diffuse loss of rod sensitivity with later cone involvement and childhood onset of night blindness. Type 2 patients showed regionalized and combined loss of rod and cone sensitivity with adult onset of night blindness.

The response of young affecteds in TCD M to two colour dark adaptometry demonstrates a greater elevation in rod sensitivity compared to cone suggesting that they would fit into Massof and Finkelstein's Type 1 category. The early age of onset would tend to confirm this.

The profile of older TCD G affecteds on the other hand shows elevation of both rod and cone thresholds but in a much more patchy pattern - some retinal loci tested having thresholds which are near normal. This would fit with a Type 2 categorization, as would the later age of onset.

Molecular genetic analysis has clearly demonstrated heterogeneity within ADRP. Clinical heterogeneity has been documented[12] even within homogenetic forms of ADRP. The definitive classification of this condition must, in all probability, await its complete molecular genetic characterization.

The author gratefully acknowledges the cooperation of members of the TCD M and TCD G kindreds in this work, and the technical assistance of Ms. Carmel Ryan and Ms. Hilary Dempsey of the Research Department of the Eye and Ear Hospital, Dublin, in performing the ERGs and of Prof. Peter Eustace and Mr. Martin Keenan of the Ophthalmology Department,

Mater Misericordiae Hospital Dublin, in carrying out two colour dark adaptometry. This work was supported by grants from the American R. P. Foundation - Fighting Blindness, R. P. Ireland - Fighting Blindness, the British R. P. Society and the Gordon Gund Foundation.

References:

1) Bradley, D., Farrar, G., Sharp, E., Kenna, P., Humphries, M., McConnell, D., Daiger, S., McWilliam, P., Humphries, P., Autosomal Dominant Retinitis Pigmentosa: Exclusion of the Gene from the Short Arm of Chromosome 1 including the Region surrounding the Rhesus Locus, Amer. J. Hum. Genet. 44; 570-576, 1989

2) Farrar, G., McWilliam, P., Sharp, E., Kenna, P., Bradley, D., Humphries, M., McConnell, D., Humphries, P., Autosomal Dominant Retinitis Pigmentosa: Exclusion of a Gene from Extensive Regions of Chromosomes 6, 13, 20, and 21 Genomics 5, 612-618, 1989

3) McWilliam, P., Farrar, G., Kenna, P., Bradley, D., Humphries, M., Sharp, E., McConnell, D., Lawler, M., Sheils, D., Ryan, C., Stevens, K., Daiger, S., Humphries, P., Autosomal Dominant Retinitis Pigmentosa (ADRP): Localization of an ADRP Gene to the Long Arm of Chromosome 3, Genomics, 5, 619-622, 1989

4) Farrar, G., McWilliam, P., Bradley, D., Kenna, P., Lawler, M., Sharp, E., Humphries, M., Eiberg, H., Conneally, M., Trofatter, J., Humphries, P., Autosomal Dominant Retinitis Pigmentosa: Linkage to Rhodopsin and Evidence for Genetic Heterogeneity, Genomics, 8, 35-40, 1990

5) Arden, G., Carter, R., Hogg, C., Powell, D., Ernst, W., Clover, G., Lyness, A., Quinlan., P., A modified ERG technique and the results obtained in X-linked retinitis pigmentosa, Br. J. Ophthalmol., 67, 419-430, 1983

6) Sondheimer, S., Fishman, G., Young, R., Vasquez, V., Dark adaptation testing in heterozygotes of Usher's syndrome, Br. J. Ophthalmol., 63, 547-550, 1979

7) Berson, E., Gouras, P., Gunkel, R., Myrianthopoulos, N., Dominant retinitis pigmentosa with reduced penetrance, Arch. Ophthalmol., 81, 226-234, 1969

8) Marmor, M., The electroretinogram in retinitis pigmentosa, Arch. Ophthalmol., 97, 1300-1304, 1979

9) Fishman, G., Alexander, K., Anderson, R., Autosomal dominant retinitis pigmentosa. A method of classification. Arch. Ophthalmol., 103, 366-374, 1985

10) Massof, R., Finkelstein, D., Two forms of autosomal dominant primary retinitis pigmentosa, Doc. Ophthalmol., 51, 289-346, 1981

11) Lyness, A., Ernst, W., Quinlan, M., Clover, G., Arden, G., Carter, R., Bird, A., Parker, J., A clinical, psychophysical, and electroretinographic survey of patients with autosomal dominant retinitis pigmentosa, Br. J. Ophthalmol., 69, 326-339, 1985

12) Berson, E., et al. In press, 1990

PROGRESS IN THE LOCALIZATION OF THE USHER SYNDROME GENES

William J. Kimberling,[1]Michael D. Weston,[1]
Sandra Pieke Dahl,[1]Yin Y. Shugart,[1]Judith B. Kenyon,[1]
Larry Overbeck,[1]Claes Moller,[2]Alessandro Martini,[3]
Richard Smith,[4]and Massimo Milani[3]

[1]Boys Town National Research Hospital; Omaha, NE
[2]University of Linkoping; Linkoping, Sweden
[3]University of Padova; Padova, Italy
[4]Baylor University; Houston, Texas

Introduction

Usher Syndrome is an autosomal recessive disorder characterized by deafness and retinitis pigmentosa (RP). Although first recognized by Von Graefe,[1]it was named after Usher[2] who emphasized its hereditary nature.

The frequency of Usher Syndrome has been estimated at 3.0/100,000 in Scandinavia and at 4.4/100,000 in the United States.[3] The prevalence of Usher Syndrome among deaf individuals has been reported to range from 0.6 to 28%.[4] Conversely, the frequency of deafness in the RP population is estimated to range between 8.0 and 33.3%. Overall, there are about 16,000 deaf and blind people in the United States, of which more than half are believed to have Usher Syndrome.

Siblings affected with Usher Syndrome are more similar with regard to clinical findings than is expected based upon the variation of symptoms in the general Usher population. This observation has led most investigators to propose that Usher Syndrome is actually two or more genetic disorders whose genes may be located at different places in the genome.[5] Type I is usually distinguishable from Type II on the basis of severity of hearing loss. Type I patients are profoundly deaf while Type II patients are 'hard of hearing.' Vestibular function seems to be a consistent discriminator between Usher Types I and II since most, if not all, type I patients completely lack vestibular function.[6]

Usher Syndrome Type II (USH2) has been recently found to be linked to locus D1S81 (pTHH33).[6,7] USH2 was placed on long arm of chromosome 1 distal to the Renin locus. The exact order of USH2 with regard to REN and D1S81 could not be established. Genetic heterogeneity of Usher Type I

(USH1) was also established since USH1 families failed to show the same 1q linkage.

This report is to: a) update the progress made towards further localization of the USH2 gene, and b) provide negative information relating to the exclusion of the USH1 gene.

Materials and Methods

Patients and Families

A total of 100 sibships with Usher Syndrome have been ascertained. There are 178 affected out of a total of 387 siblings. Of these, there are 39 type I families and 37 type II families, and 24 families which have not yet been been clinically subtyped.

Clinical Studies

Clinical studies were done at the Boys Town National Research Hospital, the University of Linkoping in Sweden, or at the University of Padova in Italy. These studies included a physical examination, an opthalmologic evaluation, standard pure tone audiometry, and a complete vestibular evaluation. The diagnosis of RP was based upon a diminished or absent ERG and a history of night blindness and peripheral field loss as well as typical fundoscopic findings. Type II Usher syndrome was diagnosed whenever a patient had an audiogram which showed a mild hearing loss in the low frequencies sloping to a profound loss in the higher frequencies, retinitis pigmentosa, and normal vestibular responses. Type I patients were defined as those with severe to profound hearing loss spanning all frequencies, retinitis pigmentosa, and absent vestibular function.

Sample Collection

Blood samples have been collected from all informative familiy members. Aliquots of blood, sera, and DNA were stored frozen for future use. Lymphoblastoid cell lines were also established.[8] Genomic DNA was extracted from whole blood or from lymphoblastoid cell lines using an Applied Biosystems DNA extraction machine.

DNA Typing

Plasmid DNA was purified following Promega Inc. technical bulletin #009. Genomic DNA was digested with appropriate restriction endonucleases, electrophoresed and blotted to charged nylon membranes (Dupont Inc.). Prepared blots were hybridized to nick-translated probes, blots were washed routinely to 0.2XSSC stringency and allowed to expose Kodak X-AR film for 1-5 days to visualize the polymorphisms.

DNA probes pEKH7.4 (D1S65), pHRnES1.9 (REN), pYNZ23 (D1S58) and pTHH33 (D1S81) were obtained thru the ATCC Human DNA Probes Repository. Table I summarizes the polymorphism information of the 4 markers used in the present linkage analysis study.[9]

TABLE 1. Polymorphism Statistics on Chromosome 1q Marker Loci Used in the Present Study

Probe	Locus	Enzyme	Allele Size (kb)	Frequency/ Heterozygosity
pEKH7.4	D1S65	TaqI	5.0	0.47
			3.8	0.53
pHRnES1.9	REN	HindIII	8.7	0.70
			6.2	0.30
pYNZ23	D1S58	MspI	5.0	0.46
			4.5	0.54
pTHH33	D1S81	RsaI	VNTR	76%

Analysis

The final linkage analysis was performed using 14 type II Usher Syndrome sibships with 82 individuals (30 affected) and 10 USH1 families with 59 individuals (24 affected). Pairwise and multipoint linkage tests and tests of locus order were performed using the MLINK, LINKMAP and ILINK options of LINKAGE 5.03. The order of the loci was assumed to be D1565-REN-D1S58-D1S81 and the recombinations between the loci were assumed to be 11, 9 and 26%, respectively. A constant sex difference of 2.1 in recombination was assumed.

Families with probands showing unusual audiograms, atypical RP, unexplained mental retardation or other neurologic disorder were excluded from the linkage analysis.[14]

Results

Two-point linkage results between USH2 and the 4 DNA markers are shown in Table 2. D1S81 gave a Z_{max} score of 7.8 at 2.0% recombination with the D1S81 locus. One obligate recombinant with D1S81 was observed in our data set. Two consanguineous marriages resulted in heterozygous affected offspring, and so two additional crossovers can be inferred although, in the analysis, this was not taken into account. The best two-point estimate places USH2 at a distance of 4.2% recombination from D1S81 with a Z_{max} of 6.5 when these additional crossovers are considered.

TABLE 2.   Two Point Lod Scores of Usher Syndrome, Type II Versus Markers on Chromosome 1q

Locus	Informative Families	Recombination fraction					
		0.00	0.01	0.05	0.10	0.20	0.30
D1S65	14	$-\infty$	-9.09	-3.70	-1.69	-0.28	0.05
REN	13	$-\infty$	-0.06	1.04	1.24	1.01	0.56
D1S58	9	$-\infty$	-0.46	1.19	1.53	1.32	0.78
D1S81	14	$-\infty$	7.71	7.52	6.69	4.68	2.58

Multipoint results which span this 1q linkage group are presented in Figure 1. The results show the USH2 gene to be slightly more likely to be proximal to the D1S81 locus.

The ILINK program was used to determine the most likely order for USH2 on the linkage group REN, D1S58 and D1S81. The relative likelihoods of the four possible orders, USH2-REN-D1S58-D1S81, REN-USH2-D1S58-D1S81, REN-D1S58-USH2-D1S81, REN-D1S58-D1S81-USH2 were $1:42:2 \times 10^5:1.3 \times 10^5$, respectively. Thus, the first two orders listed above can be dismissed. However, which side USH2 is on with respect to D1S81 can only be resolved by typing additional markers which are distal to D1S81. These markers include CRI-L744, CRI-L1191 and D1S8 (pMS32).

Table 3 shows the current status of the search for the location of the type I Usher gene. Thirty-seven loci have been studied and none show any evidence of linkage. Other investigators have also failed to find linkage with markers on other chromosomes.[11,12]

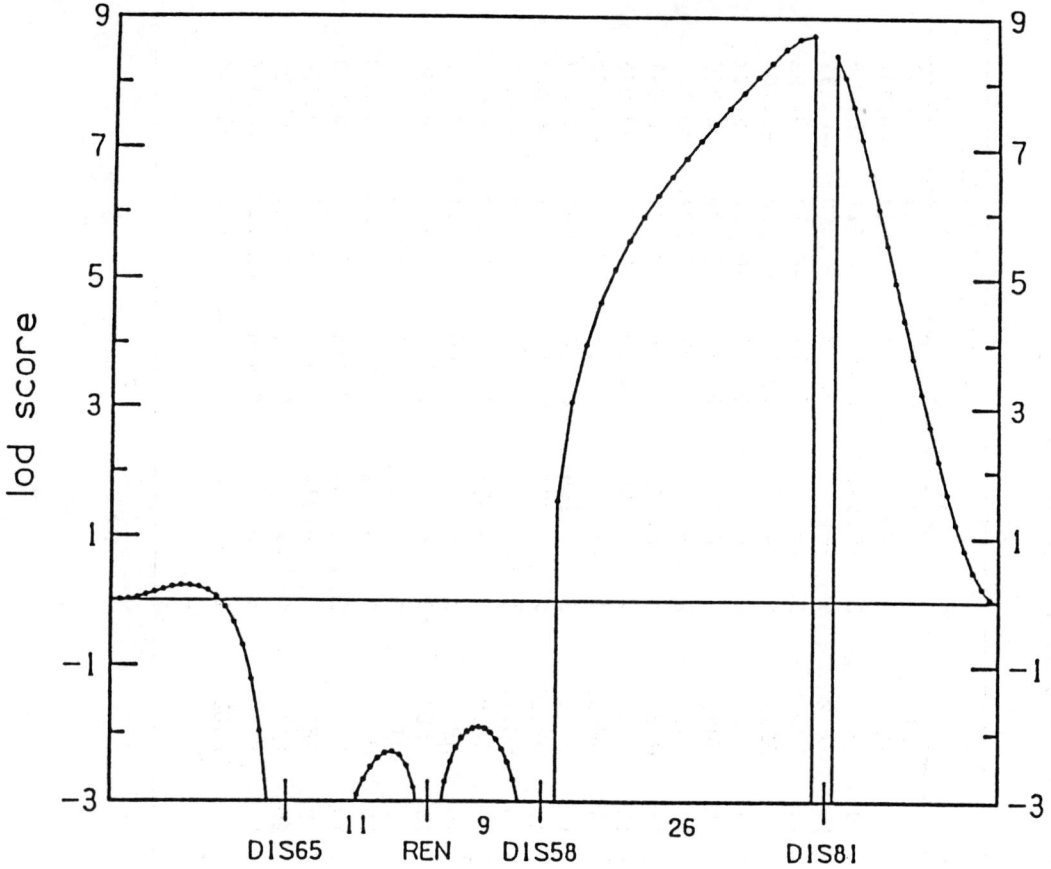

Figure 1:   Location scores for the USH2 gene on a map
defined by 4 markers from the q22 region of chromosome 1q
using LINKMAP.   The highest score (8.72) is on the
centromeric side of D1S81.   A test of order using ILINK
favors D1S58-USH2-D1S81.   However, this order is favored
only 2.0 times over the next likely alternative D1S58-D1S81-
USH2.   The map is derived from the recombination estimates
of O'Connell et al. assuming no sex difference, and scaled
in centimorgans.

Table 3.   Two Point Lod Scores of Marker Data For Usher Type I

| Chr | Locus | N | Recombination Fraction | | | | Chr | Locus | N | Recombination Fraction | | | |
			0.0	0.1	0.2	0.3				0.0	0.1	0.2	0.3
1	DR78	1	0.250	0.183	0.116	0.057	8	GPT	3	0.023	0.020	0.013	0.007
1	FY	2	-∞	-0.314	-0.110	-0.034	9	ABO	4	-∞	-0.289	-0.087	-0.021
1	H3H2	4	0.203	0.127	0.070	0.031	9	AK	2	-0.352	-0.208	-0.611	-0.048
1	NGFB	2	0.074	0.079	0.060	0.033	13	7F12	9	-∞	-0.753	-0.298	-0.133
1	PGD	1	-0.051	-0.044	-0.029	-0.014	13	ESD	3	-∞	-0.879	-0.413	-0.192
1	PGM1	4	-∞	-0.681	-0.272	-0.099	13	9D11	6	-∞	-1.580	-0.518	-0.106
1	RH	5	-∞	-0.638	-0.241	-0.084	13	1E8	4	-∞	-0.214	-0.007	0.027
1	EKH7.4	12	-∞	0.370	0.080	0.120	13	HUB8	5	0.449	0.311	0.184	0.086
1	REN	10	-∞	-0.700	-0.080	0.060	13	9A7	8	-∞	-0.007	0.201	0.122
1	L744	4	-∞	-1.200	-0.400	-0.110	13	G2E3	4	0.021	0.103	0.101	0.061
1	L1191	4	-∞	-0.220	-0.060	-0.010	13	G18E2	4	0.499	0.310	0.172	0.076
1	THH33	13	-∞	-2.630	-0.990	-0.330	14	AW101	4	-∞	-0.583	-0.259	-0.101
1	TH154	6	-∞	-0.310	0.230	0.240	14	PI	3	0.199	0.100	0.035	0.007
1	HHH106	9	-∞	-2.350	-0.920	-0.330	15	DP151	2	0.074	0.051	0.037	0.020
2	ACP	3	-0.278	-0.139	-0.060	-0.020	15	MS1-14	1	-∞	-0.210	-0.054	-0.010
3	TNF	2	0.250	0.166	0.096	0.044	16	3HVR	1	-0.051	-0.044	-0.029	-0.014
3	B67	5	-∞	-1.280	-0.51	-0.160	16	HP	3	-∞	-0.146	-0.011	-0.011
3	EFD145	13	-∞	-0.610	0.020	0.100	16	EKD2	13	-∞	-0.004	0.390	0.280
3	MCT32	10	-∞	-1.970	-0.650	-0.210	18	JK	3	-0.102	0.000	0.024	0.018
3	TNF	5	-∞	-1.380	-0.650	-0.280	19	C3	2	0.375	0.267	0.165	0.079
3	YNZ86	11	-∞	0.630	0.500	0.280	19	LE	5	-0.087	-0.054	-0.029	-0.013
3	H3H2	10	-∞	-0.230	0.110	0.100	19	SEC	5	0.074	0.054	0.033	0.016
4	GC	1	-0.352	-0.191	-0.097	-0.040	20	ADA	2	-∞	-0.580	-0.267	-0.107
4	MNS	5	-0.029	0.050	0.053	0.032	22	P1	4	-∞	-0.538	-0.242	-0.096
6	BF	1	0.125	0.084	0.049	0.023	?	KELL	1	-0.176	-0.104	-0.056	-0.024
6	GLO	4	0.625	0.521	0.357	0.186							

N_s = # of informative families.

Discussion

An example of clinical application of the USH2 linkage has yet to be reported. The linkage has an obvious use in early diagnosis of at risk infants. Heterozygote detection of sibs and other relatives is possible, but is of limited value since there is as yet no means of carrier detection for the potential mates of Usher family members. By virtue of the fact that the linkage can determine heterozygotes, it is now possible to resolve the issue of heterozygote expression of the USH2 gene. Also, the localization has the potential of clarifying the diagnosis of phenotypically confusing families. For example, are families with progressive hearing loss and RP a variant of type 2 or are they genetically distinct?

The localization of the Usher Syndrome Type 2 gene is a significant step forward to eventually cloning this gene. The exact position of the USH2 gene is currently being actively pursued in our laboratory. New probes in the 1q region are being tested in an effort to define a pair of markers that flank the USH2 gene.

References

1. Von Graefe, A. (1858). Vereinzelte Beobachtungen und Bernerkunger: Exceptionelles Verhalten des Gesichtfeldes bei Pigmententartung der Netzhaut. Von Graefe's Arch. Ophthal. 4: 250-253.
2. Usher, C. H. (1935). The Bowman lecture: On a few hereditary eye afflictions. Trans. Ophtal. Soc. UK 55:164.
3. Hallgren, B. (1959). Retinitis pigmentosa combined with congenital deafness; with vestibulo-cerebellar ataxia and mental abnormality in a proportion of cases. A clinical and genetico-statistical study. Acad. Psychiatr. Scand. (Suppl.) 138:5-101.
4. Boughman, J. A., Vernon, M., Shaver, K. A. (1983). Usher syndrome: Definition and estimate of prevalence from two high-risk populations. J. Chron. Dis. 36:595-603.
5. Moller, C. G., Kimberling, W. J., Davenport, S. L. H., Priluck, I., White, V., Biscone-Halterman, K., Odkvist, L., Brookhouser, P.E., Lund, G. and Grissom, T. J. (1989). Usher syndrome: An otoneurologic study. Laryngoscope 99:73-79.
6. Kimberling, W. J., Moller, C. G., Davenport, S. L. H., Lund, G., Grissom, T. J., Priluck, I., White, V., Weston, M. D., Biscone-Halterman, K. A. and Brookhouser, P. E. (1989). Usher syndrome: Clinical findings and gene localization studies. Laryngoscope 99:66-72.

7. Lewis, R. A., Otterud, B., Stauffer, D., Lalouel, J. M., and Leppert, M. (1989). Mapping recessive ophthalmic diseases: Linkage of the locus for Usher syndrome type II to a DNA marker on chromosome 1q. Genomics 7:250-256.

8. Neitzel, H. (1986). A routine method for the establishment of permanent growing lymphoblastoid cell lines. Hum. Genet. 73:320-326.

9. O'Connell, P., Lathrop, G. M., Nakamura, Y., Leppert, M. L., Ardinger, R. H., Murray, J. L., Lalouel, J. M., and White, R. (1989). Twenty eight loci form a continuous linkage map of markers for human chromosome 1. *Genomics* 4:12-20.

10. Kimberling, W. J. Moller, C. G., Davenport, S. L. H., Lund, G., Grissom, T. J., Priluck, I., White, V., Weston, M. D., Biscone-Halterman, K. A. and Brookhouser, P. E. (1989). Usher syndrome: Clinical findings and gene localization studies. *Laryngoscope* 99:66-72.

11. Pelias, M. Z., Lemoine, D. R., Kossar, A. L., Ward, L. J., Wilson, A. F., Elston, R. C. (1988). Linkage studies of Usher syndrome : Analysis of an Acadian kindred in Louisiana. Cytogenet. Cell Genet. 47:111-112.

12. Smith, R. J. H., Holcomb, J. D., Daiger, S. P., Caskey, C. T., Pelias, M. Z., Alford, B. R., et al. (1989). The exclusion of Usher syndrome gene from much of chromosome 4. *Cytogenet. Cell Genet.* 50:102-106.

AN APPROACH TO CLONING THE PROXIMAL LOCUS FOR X-LINKED RETINITIS PIGMENTOSA

Susan Riley , Graeme Black, Zhengyi Chen, Eli Hatchwell, Birgit Lorenz[2], Thomas Meitinger[1], John Powell, Baerbel Wittwer[3] and Ian Craig

The Genetics Laboratory, Department of Biochemistry, University of Oxford and [1]Abteilung fur paediatrische Genetik, Kinderpoliklinik der Universitaet Muenchen. [2]Augenklinik der Universitaet Muenchen. [3]Institut fuer medizinische Genetik am Bezirkskrankenhaus Magdeburg.

INTRODUCTION

Among the range of apparently similar forms of inherited retinal degeneration, X-linked retinitis pigmentosa is one of the most severe. Several recent investigations have suggested that the X-linked form of the disorder may be genetically heterogeneous although it has not been possible to distinguish separate types clinically. An understanding of the probable existence of heterogeneity in the X-linked disorder has emerged with the increasing information made available from genetic analysis[1-5] coupled with the information from a patient manifesting a multiple disorder syndrome including retinitis pigmentosa and a deletion of parts of Xp21 and p11.4 [6]. The available data are consistent with the existence of (at least) two RP loci, one close to OTC (ie distal to DXS7) and the other proximal to DXS7.

We have previously reported on the use of the probe M27beta which detects the hypervariable locus DXS255 in the analysis of several German pedigrees[7]. No recombination was observed in 4 families representing 17 informative meioses, but 2 recombinants in 12 meioses were seen in an additional family. Further studies with this probe[8,9] have shown close linkage to the disease locus in some larger XLRP families and suggest a proximal location for the RP gene in a proportion of the pedigrees examined. M27beta therefore represents a valuable genetic marker in assessing heterogeneity and, in combination with DXS426, a recently introduced microsatellite marker[9,10], provides good evidence for the existence of a second X-linked gene involved in the aetiology of retinitis pigmentosa mapping in the vicinity of these two marker loci.

Isolation and characterisation of genes for genetic disorders can follow from molecular investigation of chromosome translocations, or deletions, which disrupt, or eliminate, the coding sequences involved. This approach may be appropriate for the more distal locus (RP3), which is probably included in the deletion with multiple disorders described above. There are no known chromosomal rearrangements in the vicinity of the second, proximal locus, RP2, resulting in the manifestation of X-linked RP. In this case, isolation of candidate genes will depend on accurate genetic mapping coupled with the establishment of a physical map and the isolation of overlapping contiguous genomic clones for the target region. To this end, we are developing a range of molecular reagents for genetic and physical mapping in the region Xp11.22 (defined by DXS255) to Xp11.4/11.3 (defined by DXS7). Our strategy is based on the amplification of sequences from hybrids retaining human X-chromosomal fragments in the appropriate region and developing these for application in genetic and physical mapping. We are also developing a range of markers based on the microsatellite (AC)n repeats, which we have isolated from within the monoamine oxidase-A locus; this has been mapped in our laboratory by in situ hybridisation with a peak of grains over the mid-point of the interval Xp11.23-p11.4[11] and is in very close proximity to Ll.28 (DXS7)[12,13].

MATERIALS AND METHODS

PREPARATION OF IRRADIATED TRANSFERRANT HYBRIDS

Cl2D, which is a human-hamster hybrid cell-line containing a single human X chromosome, was gamma irradiated and fused with a hamster cell line (A23) as described by Benham et al[14] employing a dosage of 50,000 rads. The clones were isolated, one per culture dish, and, following the freezing down of early passage material, DNA preparations were made and distributed to the various centres involved in their preliminary characterisation (Goodfellow et al in preparation). The presence/absence of sequences corresponding to 8 short arm probes and 18 long arm probes was ascertained for >200 clones by Southern blotting to provide preliminary information on the hybrids; however, not all hybrids were examined for the full repertoire of long arm probes.   A subgroup of hybrids were chosen for more detailed analysis with additional, proximal short arm probes.   Dr M. Coleman, Institute of Molecular Medicine also tested a selection of these for the presence of DXS426 by the polymerase chain reaction as described previously[9]. The proximal short arm probes employed in the combined analysis were: DXS7, DXS255, DXS146, DXS14, DXS34 and DXS90. All of these are described by Mandel et al[15]. In addition, we employed IB/D22 kindly provided by John Cowell (C.R.C. London).

FAMILY STUDIES/RFLP ANALYSIS AND LINKAGE STUDIES

The criteria for diagnosis of X-linked RP, examination of RFLPs and linkage analysis were as described previously[7].

POLYMERASE CHAIN REACTION

Alu amplification of human sequences from irradiated fragment hybrids followed the procedure described by Nelson et al[16] with slight modifications (annealing temperature 68°, and 20 ng DNA per reaction). PCR analysis of the DXS426 locus in the German pedigrees was performed as described by Coleman et al[9]. Products were analysed on 6% polyacrylamide gels and visualised with silver staining reagents (Biorad Ltd).

RESULTS

ANALYSIS OF GERMAN RP PEDIGREES WITH HYPERVARIABLE PROBES DXS426 AND DXS255

We applied the PCR based analysis of variable alleles at the DXS426 locus to the families described previously[7]. Three additional families were analysed with both DXS255 and DXS426. 41 meioses were informative for M27beta and RP and of these 33 were informative for both probes. In total, we observed 58 meiosis informative for both DXS255 and DXS426 without observing any recombinants. There were 5 cross-overs between RP and DXS426 which were also recombinant for DXS255 (see TABLE 1).

TABLE 1
Lod Scores of the Linkage Analysis between M27beta and Retinitis Pigmentosa

pedigree	meioses	recombinants	Zmax(theta)
01	12	2	1.2 (0.15)
02	3	0	0.9 (0.0)
03	4	0	1.0 (0.0)
04	6	0	1.6 (0.0)
05	4	0	1.0 (0.0)
06	2	0	-
07	2	0	-
08	12	3	0.7 (0.25)

DEVELOPMENT OF NEW GENETIC MARKERS BASED ON GENOMIC CLONES IN THE MONOAMINE OXIDASE-A (MAO) REGION

MAO exists as two genetically distinct forms MAO-A and MAO-B. The two genes map very close to each other on the proximal short arm of the human X-chromosome (see Levy et al.[11]). Our survey of 8 lambda phage clones containing genomic sequences with MAO coding sequences detected three (AC)n repeat regions. We have designated these MAO/AC1,2 (from the mid region of the gene) & MAO/AC3 (close to the 5' end). Oligonucleotides were prepared corresponding to flanking sequences for two of these and have been demonstrated to amplify, by the polymerase chain reaction, variable alleles at significant frequency. Examples of the analysis of the PCR products for MAO/AC1 (primers 1 & 2) are illustrated in Figure 1. Primers 1 and 2 detect five alleles, three of which are prevalent (see TABLE 2).

Two bands separated by about 6 bp are observed for most alleles with the slower migrating band of stronger intensity. Heterozygotes generally show four bands eg individuals 43 and 49 (Figure 1). Examination of the progeny of 43, a manifesting carrier, suggest that her daughter, 42, should also be a carrier, unless a cross-over has occurred. An identical conclusion was reached on previous analysis with M27beta[7]; subsequent clinical investigation has confirmed her carrier status. Preliminary observations with MAO/AC2 (primers 3 and 4) suggests a lower level of heterogeneity. MAO/AC3 remains to be tested.

TABLE 2
Allele Frequencies Detected with MAO (AC)n Repeat I Primers
(MAO 1 and 2)

	Approx size (bp)	Frequency
Allele A	112	0.44
Allele B	114	0.30
Allele C	116	0.01
Allele D	118	0.24
Allele E	122	0.01

24 females and 32 males representing 6 families and 4 unrelated
individuals were examined
Calculated heterozygosity   = 0.66
Observed heterozygosity   = 0.30

The application of a combined PCR approach to the analysis of the three
(AC)n repeat regions in the MAO-A gene should provide additional
information to that provided by LI.28, as DXS7 and the MAO-A and -B loci
are very close[13]. Long range restriction mapping results place the MAO loci
within 1.2 Mb of DXS7[12,17]. It should now be possible to detect crossovers
between the region including these markers (LI.28 and MAO) and RP2 in a
significantly greater number of meioses than hitherto possible.

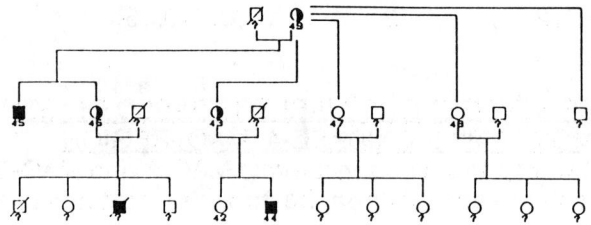

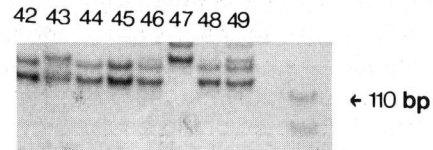

42 43 44 45 46 47 48 49

← 110 bp

KEY:
○ – Normal ♀   ◑ – Carrier ♀
□ – Normal ♂   ■ – Affected ♂
⊘ ⊠ – Deceased
? – Sample not available

Figure 1   PCR products obtained with MAO (AC)n Repeat I Primers
(MAO 1 and 2)

IRRADIATION FRAGMENT HYBRIDS AS AN ENRICHED SOURCE OF PROBES FOR THE REGION EMBRACING RP2

The original panel of irradiation fragment hybrids was derived from a human/hamster hybrid retaining the X chromosome as its only genetic material (see Materials and Methods). 224 different clones were examined in a multicentre programme for a range of X-chromosomal markers including 18 long arm probes and 8 short arm probes. From these, we selected 50 hybrid lines containing at least one marker within the proximal X short arm region Xp11.4-Xcen for a more detailed investigation with additional markers (see Materials and Methods). After eliminating hybrids with large inserts, or with apparently complex retention patterns, a subpanel of X hybrids was chosen for evaluation by PCR amplification of human genomic material (TABLE 3). Of the hybrids finally selected, most retained X-chromsomal fragments of between 3-10 Mb. Where the order of probes was not unequivocally established previously, that consistent with the fewest breakpoints was assumed. Use of polymerase chain reactions employing *Alu* sequence primers similar to those described by Nelson et al[16] resulted in the amplification of discrete fragments in the size range 400bp - 5kb for several hybrids. Cloning of PCR products into pUC9 yielded recombinant plasmids with a wide range of inserts (Figure 2).

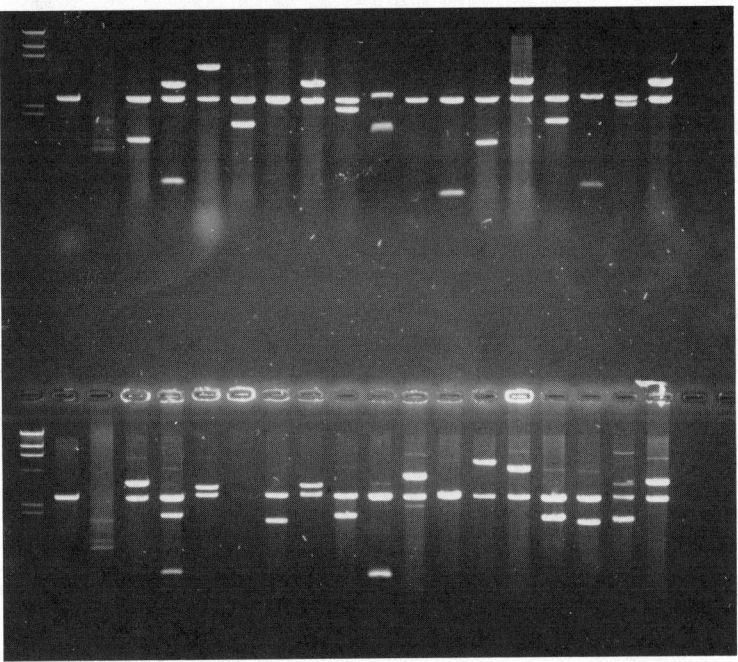

Figure 2   The range of inserts obtained following cloning of *Alu* primed PCR products from hybrid 81. Track 1-3 of both upper and lower series contain standards [track1 - HindIII lambda marker; track 2 - vector alone; track 3 - total PCR product]. Inserts released by digestion with appropriate restriction enzyme.

TABLE 3

Distribution of X-short arm Probes in various Irradiation Fragment Hybrids

CELL REF	DXS7 L1.28	DXS426 (AC)n	DXS255 M27beta	DXS146 PTAK8	DXS14 P58-1	IB/D22	DXS34 RD-6	DXS90 PXG-20
17/7/01	1	?	ND	0	0	ND	ND	0
17/7/02	1	0	1	0	1	ND	ND	0
17/7/03	1	0	0	1	0	0	0	0
17/7/04	1	0	1	1	0	0	0	2
17/7/05 $	2	ND	1	0	1	2	0	0
17/7/06	2	1	0	2	0	1	0	0
17/7/07	0	ND	1	0	0	0	0	0
17/7/08	0	ND	2	2	1	0	0	0
17/7/09	0	ND	0	2	0	1	0	0
17/7/10 *	0	0	0	2	1	0	0	0
17/7/11	0	ND	0	0	1	1	0	0
17/7/12	0	ND	0	0	2	1	0	0
17/7/13	0	ND	0	0	1	0	0	0
17/7/14	0	ND	0	0	1	ND	1	0
17/7/15	0	ND	0	0	0	0	1	0

*   STS present
$ Pseudoautosomal (DXYS20) present
Single long arm probes detected in 05,11 & 14
Where intermediate probes have not been tested, contiguity is assumed (hybrid 14)
Centromeric (DXZ1) sequences are retained in all except 08, 14 & 15
1 = strong signal; 2 = weak signal; ND = Not Determined

Several of the inserts are of similar size to major bands observed in the total PCR products. They do not appear to represent highly repetitive sequences as most of the inserts do not hybridise to total human DNA (37/40); neither do they appear to be hamster contaminants as only three inserts were significantly labelled following hybridization with total hamster DNA.

We have taken several clones and demonstrated their potential as useful X-chromosome genetic markers by hybridising their inserts to panels of DNA samples from males, females and a range of somatic cell hybrids (eg human X-only hybrid line Thy BX - shown in Figure 3). X-specificity is indicated by dosage in male and female tracks and by a signal in the X-only hybrid lane (see arrow c. 7kb).

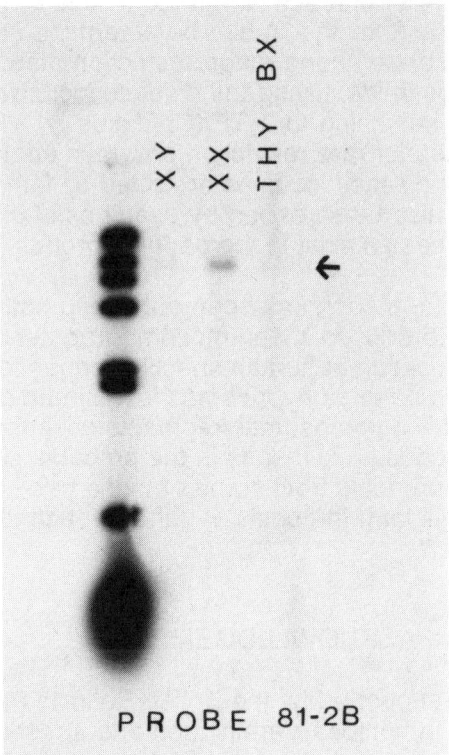

Figure 3 Southern blot of genomic DNA probed with labelled clone 81-A and illustrating X specificity from dosage (left hand track = HindIII lambda marker).   No hybridisation was observed to mouse or hamster genomic DNA (not shown).

DISCUSSION

Our data indicate the close linkage of DXS255 and DXS426 and add support to the existence of two RP loci; one closely linked to these two loci and the other at a considerable distance. It is difficult without large pedigrees to conclude for any one family whether or not the proximal or distal locus is involved; however, the availability of additional highly informative probes in the mid-region between the two would greatly facilitate the distinction between RP2 and RP3. In addition, we have pointed out that a strategy for the isolation of candidate genes for the proximal X-linked retinitis locus (RP2) will require accurate pinpointing of the disorder through analysis of individual cross-overs in carrier females multiply informative for a range of proximal short arm probes. Isolation and development of such probes is now possible through the approach of amplifying DNA segments for the desired region which in turn can be used to isolate genomic DNA containing (AC)n repeats. Such repeats are frequently distributed in the genome; indeed, we have described the existence of three such sequences within 40kb of the monoamine oxidase A gene. It follows that the strategy of isolating X chromosomal sequences from the target region and employing these to subsequently isolate cosmids or YACs, which can then be screened for (AC)n repeats should be of considerable assistance in progress to this goal. One advantage of this approach is that it provides a ready supply of sequences whose genetic relationship can be determined and which can also be employed to generate a long range restriction map.

The subsequent steps in identifying the disease locus would follow the well established path of searching for HTF (CpG-cluster) islands which appear as clusters of sites for rare restriction enzymes on the long range map in the vicinity of the disease locus as predicted by family studies. Candidate genes could also be screened by searches of cDNA libraries with such conserved sequences as exist in the panel of probes isolated for the target zone.

The feasibility of this approach has been enhanced both through the availability of irradiation produced X chromosome fragment hybrids and the technique of PCR amplification of human specific sequences from these. Our analysis of one such panel of hybrids has identified a range of clones which retain a variety of X-chromosomal fragments covering the region Xcen to Xp11.4. Several hybrids have inserts in the probable size range 2-5 Mb. Cloning of human PCR products from some of these has provided valuable source material which will form the basis of our approach to cloning the RP2 locus.

ACKNOWLEDGEMENTS

This study was partially supported by the British Retinitis Pigmentosa Society, the Deutsche Retinitis Pigmentosa-Vereinigung and a research grant to T.M. by the Deutsche Forschungsgemeinschaft. Eli Hatchwell is a Wellcome Clinical Research Fellow. We thank C. Doerner and E. Strobach for expert technical assistance.

REFERENCES

1.   Wright, A.F., Bhattacharya, S., Clayton, J.F., Dempster, M., Tippett, P., McKeown, C.M., Jay, M. and Bird, A.C., Linkage relationships between X-linked retinitis pigmentosa and nine short arm markers: exclusion of the disease locus from Xp21 and localisation between DXS7 and DXS14, Am J. Hum. Genet. 41, 635, 1988.

2.   Musarella, MA, Argonza, R., Burghes, A., Kim, G., Tsui, L-C. and Worton, R.G., Linkage analysis of X-linked retinitis pigmentosa (RP2), Cytogenet. Cell Genet. 46, 666, 1987.

3. Wirth, B., Denton, M.J. Chen, J-D. Neugebauer, M., Halliday, F.B., van Schooneveld, M., Donald, J., Bleeker-Wagemakers, E.M., Pearson, P.L. and Gal, A., Two diferent genes for X-linked retinitis pigmentosa, <u>Genomics</u> 2, 263, 1988

4. Chen, J.D. Dickinson, P., Gray, R., Constable, I., Sheffield, L. and Denton, M.J., Non-allelic mutations in X-linked retinitis pigmentosa, <u>Clinical Genetics</u> 35, 338, 1989.

5. Ott, J., Bhattacharya, S., Chen, J.D., Denton, M.J., Donal, J., Dubay, C., Faffar, G.J. Fishman, G., Frey, D., Gal A., Humphries, P., Jay, B., Jay, M., Macchler, M., Musarella, M., Neugebauer, M., Nussbaum, R.L. Terwilliger, J.D., Weleber, R.G., Wirth, B., Wong, F., Worton, R.G. and Wright, A., Localizing multiple X-chromosome-linked retinitis pigmentosa loci using multilocus homogeneity tests, <u>Proc. Natl. Acad. Sci. USA.</u> 87, 701, 1990.

6. Francke, U. Ochs, H.D., de Martinville, B., Giacalone, J., Lingren, V., Disteche, C., Pagon, R.A. Hofker, M.H. van Ommen, G-J. B., Pearson,. P.L. and Wedgewood, R.J., Minor Xp21 chromosome deletion in a male associated with expression of Duchenne muscular dystrophy, chronic granulamatomous disease, retinitis pigmentosa and McLeod syndrome.
<u>Am. J. Hum. Genet.</u> 37, 250, 1985.

7. Meitinger, T., Fraser, N.J., Lorenz, B., Zrenner, E., Murken, J. and Craig, I.W., Linkage of X-linked retinitis pigmentosa to the hypervariable DNA marker M27beta (DXS255).
<u>Hum. Genet.</u> 81, 283, 1989.

8. Wright, A.F., Bhattacharya, S., Jay, M., Carothers, A.D., Bird, A.C., Jay, B. and Evans, H., Heterogeneity in X-linked retinitis pigmentosa.
<u>Cytogenet Cell Genet</u>. 51, 1110, 1989.

9. Coleman, M, Bhattacharya, S., Lindsay, S., Wright, A., Jay, M., Litt, M., Craig, I. and Davies, K., Localisation of the microsatellite probe DXS426 between DXS7 and DXS255 on Xp and linkage to retinitis pigmentosa, <u>Am. J. Hum. Genet.</u>,
1990 in press.

10. Luty, J.A., Willard, H.F. and Litt, M. ,Three new microsatellite VNTRs on the X chromsome,
<u>Cytogenet Cell Genet.</u> 51, 1036, 1989.

11. Levy, E.R. Powell, J.F., Buckle, V.J., Hsu, Y-P.P., Breakefield, X.O., and Craig, I.W., Localisation of human monoamine oxidase-A gene to Xp11.23-11.4 by <u>in situ</u> hybridisation: implications for Norrie disease, <u>Genomics</u> 5, 368, 1989.

12. Diergaarde, P.J., Weiringa, B., Bleeker-Wagemakers, E.M., Sims, K.B., Breakefield, X.O. and Ropers, H-H., Physical fine mapping of a deletion spanning the Norrie gene, <u>Hum. Genet.</u> 84, 22, 1989

13. Sims, K.B., de la Chapelle, A., Norio, R., Sankila, E.-M., Hsu, Y-P.P., Rinehart, W.B., Corey, T.J., Ozelius, L., Powell, J.F., Bruns, G., Gusella, J.F., Murphy, D.L. and Breakefield, X.O., Monoamine oxidase deficiency in males with an X-chromosome deletion, <u>Neurone</u> 2, 1069, 1989.

14. Benham, F., Hart, K., Crolla, J., Bobrow, M., Francavilla, M. and Goodfellow, P.N., A method for generating hybrids containing nonselected fragments of human chromsomes, <u>Genomics</u> 4, 509,1989.

15. Mandel, J-L, Willard, H.F., Nussbaum, R.L., Romeo, G., Puck, J.M. and Davies, K.E., Report of the committee on the genetic constitution of the X-chromosome. (HGM10 1989), <u>Cytogenet Cell Genet.</u> 51, 384, 1989.

16. Nelson, D.L., Ledbetter, S.A., Corbo, L., Victoria, M.F., Ramirez-Solis, R., Webster, T.D., Ledbetter, D.H. and Caskey, T., *Alu* polymerase chain reaction: A method for rapid isolation of human-specific sequences from complex DNA sources, <u>Proc. Natl. Acad Sci. USA</u> 86, 6686, 1989.

17. Chen, Z-Y., Powell, J.F. Breakefield, X.O. and Craig, I.W. unpublished data, 1990.

XLRP (RP3): FURTHER LINKAGE DATA, PHYSICAL MAPPING OF TWO DNA MARKERS CLOSELY LINKED TO RP3 BY PULSED FIELD GEL ELECTROPHORESIS AND CLONING STRATEGIES

MARIA A. MUSARELLA,[1,2] CATHY MCDOWELL,[1] C. LYNN ANSON-CARTWRIGHT,[1] ARTHUR H.M. BURGHES,[3] AND JOHANNA M. ROMMENS[1]

1. DEPARTMENT OF GENETICS, THE RESEARCH INSTITUTE, HOSPITAL FOR SICK CHILDREN, TORONTO, ONTARIO, CANADA 2. DEPARTMENT OF OPHTHALMOLOGY, HOSPITAL FOR SICK CHILDREN, TORONTO, ONTARIO, CANADA 3. DEPARTMENTS OF MOLECULAR GENETICS, PHYSIOLOGICAL CHEMISTRY AND NEUROLOGY, UNIVERSITY OF OHIO, COLUMBUS, OHIO, U.S.A.

I. INTRODUCTION

The most severe clinical form of retinitis pigmentosa (RP) is the X-linked type (XLRP) in which blindness occurs by the third or fourth decade of life. About 1 in 20,000 individuals are affected. Although decades of research into the biochemistry and physiology of this disease have failed to elucidate the defect, considerable excitement has recently been generated by the potential of the application of "reverse genetics" to this problem. In this approach a gene is identified by its chromosomal position rather than by its function.[1,2] The power of this approach has been demonstrated in the successful identification of genes which when defective result in chronic granulomatous disease,[3] Duchenne muscular dystrophy,[4,5] retinoblastoma[6] and cystic fibrosis.[7]

Using "reverse genetics" to localize the gene involved in a disease requires one to move from a primary genetic map generated by linkage analysis to a physical map which delimits the DNA region containing the gene. XLRP was initially mapped to the Xp11 region.[8] This locus has been designated RP2. Further studies have detected another XLRP locus (RP3) at Xp21 close to OTC.[9-13] The RP3 locus is found in approximately 75% of XLRP families.[14] In this paper we review the current status of genetic linkage studies for RP3, present a long-range physical map generated with two DNA markers closely linked to the RP3 locus and discuss the stategies we are using to isolate the RP3 gene.

II. LOCALIZING THE RP3 GENE

A. LINKAGE ANALYSIS ON FAMILIES WITH XLRP

Lod score values from eighteen XLRP families were calculated using various values of recombination distances, θ, for each locus tested. For these families (two families were given to us by Dr. R. Nussbaum, eight families are from Dr. G.H. Fishman) XLRP was found to be tightly linked to two genetic markers in Xp21, OTC and DXS84 (754), with a θ_{max} of 0.04 (LOD = 13.65) (95% confidence limits of $\theta = 0.0001$-0.11) and 0.04 (LOD =7.99) (95% confidence limit of $\theta = 0.0004$ - 0.18), respectively. RFLP locus DXS206 (XJ), also shows linkage to XLRP with a $\theta_{max} = 0.04$ (LOD = 4.57). Polymorphic probes involving the Xp11- Xcen region are distantly related to the XLRP gene.

With the hypervariable probe DXS255 (M27β), which is mapped to Xp11-Xcen, θ_{max} is 0.20 (LOD = 5.75) and for DXS7 (L1.28), mapping to Xp11.3, θ_{max} is 0.13 (LOD = 6.20). Data from recombinations in these families places the locus for XLRP above OTC and below DXS141 (pERT145-12) consistent with an Xp21 localization. In one family one of the affected males has an apparent recombination between XLRP and all markers tested except for DXS28 (C7) suggesting that in this single family the XLRP mutation maps near DXS28 and above the DMD gene markers.

Multilocus analysis was performed on all families in order to position XLRP relative to other loci. Using the ILINK program the relative odds in favor of the order XLRP-754-OTC-L1.28 is 3.50×10^5 times more likely than the order 754-OTC-L1.28-XLRP. Although the order 754-XLRP-OTC-L1.28 is 10 times less likely than XLRP-754-OTC-L1.28, the difference is not significant. Multipoint linkage analysis was also done using the LINKAGE 5.03 (linkmap) program.[15] This analysis allows multipoint lod scores to be derived by moving the disease locus between the markers and calculating the lod score for a given map distance. Each map consists of overlapping maps of three or four marker loci and the disease locus. Under the hypothesis of homogeneity, the location of the XLRP locus was found at a map distance of 2.5 cM distal to OTC (RP3). The maximum lod score at this map distance is 53.29. Testing under the alternate hypothesis of heterogeneity provides evidence for two XLRP loci that are linked. One locus is 6 cM distal to DXS164 (pERT 87-15) and the other is 1.2 cM distal to OTC. Testing heterogeneity against homogeneity gives an odds ratio of 15:1 in favor of a second disease locus, most likely located between DXS28 and DXS164 near the Duchenne muscular dystrophy locus. Further heterogeneity testing for 3 disease loci failed to detect a third XLRP locus proximal to DXS7 in any of our XLRP families.[16]

B. PHYSICAL STUDIES: Xp21 DELETION PATIENTS

The genetic localization of RP3 to Xp21is supported by the analysis of Xp21 deletions found in two male patients, BB and SB, with multiple disease phenotypes. BB had four X-linked disorders: chronic granulomatous disease (CGD), DMD, McLeod phenotype (XK) and retinitis pigmentosa (RP);[17] SB had CGD, McLeod phenotype and RP.[18] Molecular analysis and pulsed-field gel electrophoresis (PFGE) mapping of these two deletions relative to other Xp21 deletions in which the RP phenotype is not present supports the relative ordering of probes and gene loci shown in Figure 1.[19-21] Based on these results the RP3 locus is positioned in the most proximal region of the DNA deleted in BB, flanked by the centromeric deletion breakpoint in BB and the CGD locus.[20]

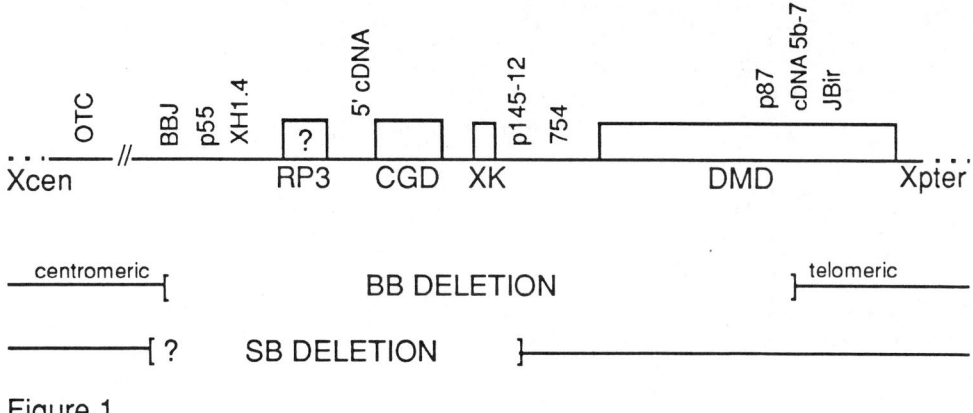

Figure 1

III. CLONING OF THE BB JUNCTION

The telomeric endpoint of the deletion in BB has been mapped between DXS240 (J-BIR) and DXS164 (pERT87-15) within the DMD gene[22] (Figure 1). We used DMD cDNA probes to detect and clone an altered size restriction fragment containing the BB deletion breakpoint. The DMD cDNA probe 5b-7 (containing exons lying between DXS240 and DXS164) was used to screen a series of restriction enzyme digests of BB genomic DNA. Novel junction fragments are generated in the DNA of individuals carrying a deletion chromosome by the joining of the deletion endpoints. Using the probe EP.9 (a 950 bp EcoRI +PstI fragment of 5b-7), we detected an 18 kb HindIII restriction fragment in a digest of genomic DNA from a normal individual, but a 10 kb band was detected in the HindIII digest of BB DNA (Figure 2, step 1).

The altered HindIII fragment was isolated from a size-selected BB genomic DNA library constructed in the phage vector, λ DASH. BB DNA, isolated from a lymphoblastoid cell line, was digested with HindIII to completion and size-fractionated by preparative agarose gel electrophoresis. DNA fragments in the size range of 8-12 kb were excised from the gel and purified by electroelution. These DNA sequences were ligated to the HindIII digested phage arms of λ DASH (insert range 9-22 kb), packaged and plated. This library, enriched for 10 kb HindIII fragments, was screened with EP.9 (Figure 2, step 2) and a phage clone containing a single 10 kb HindIII insert was purified: BBJ-1. The identity of BBJ-1 was confirmed by rehybridization of this sequence to the same Southern blot in which the BB junction fragment was originally detected. BB genomic DNA showed the same 10 kb HindIII band seen initially. In the normal individual the original 18 kb fragment was detected, as well as a new 5 kb HindIII fragment (Figure 2, step 3).

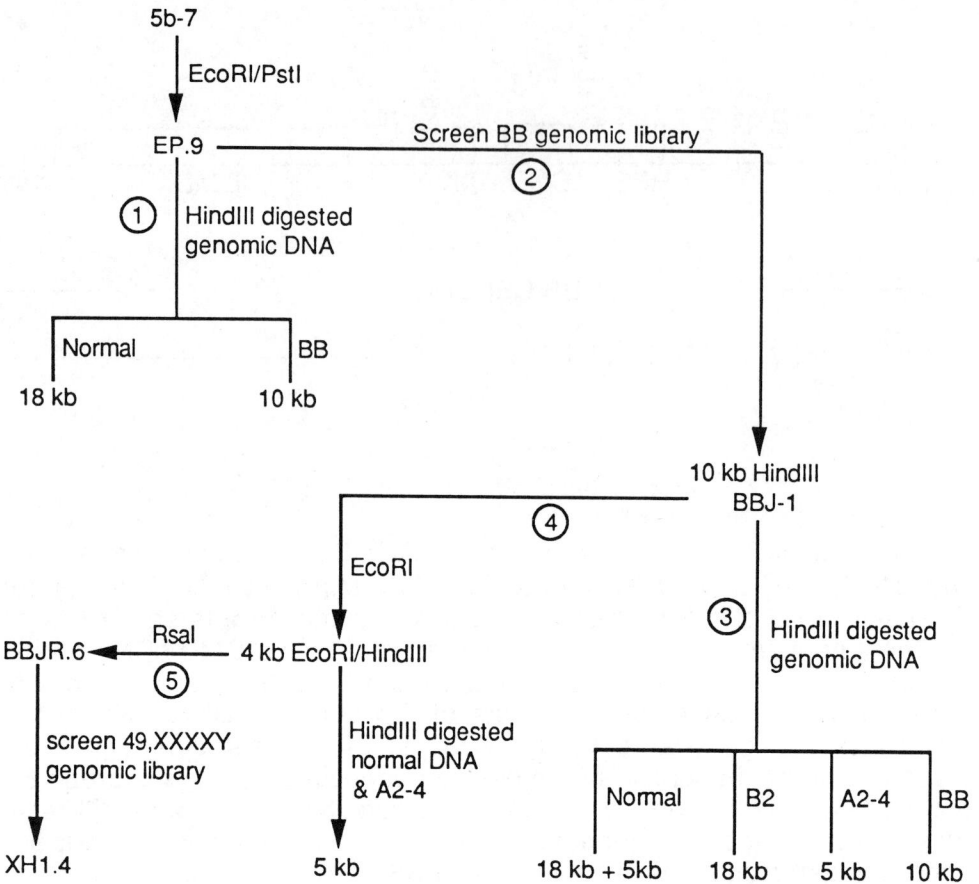

Figure 2

The cloned insert contains DNA flanking the BB deletion breakpoint from the centromeric and telomeric sides. Hybrid cell lines were used to position sequences from the BB junction clone in the Xp21 region. Two mouse:human somatic cell hybrids containing the human derivative chromosomes resulting from a (X;21) translocation were crucial for mapping sequences from the BBJ-1 insert to the centromeric or telomeric side of the deletion breakpont. The t(X;21) breakpoint mapped to the DMD gene between exons 7 and 8.[23] These DMD exons are in the region of DNA deleted in BB. The cell line A2-4 contains the derivative X chromosome and has all human X chromosome sequences proximal to the translocation breakpoint. The derivative chromosome 21 is present in the cell line B2 which therefore contains only the human X chromosome DNA extending from the distal side of the translocation breakpoint to the telomere. Since the translocation breakpoint is located within the BB deletion, the pieces of the X chromosome isolated in these two cell lines effectively separate the centromeric and telomeric sequences of the junction clone. A schematic representation of the translocation event is shown in Figure 3. Therefore, DNA sequences from the centromeric side of the BB deletion breakpoint hybridized only to A2-4 (derX), whereas distal sequences hybridized to B2 (der2l).

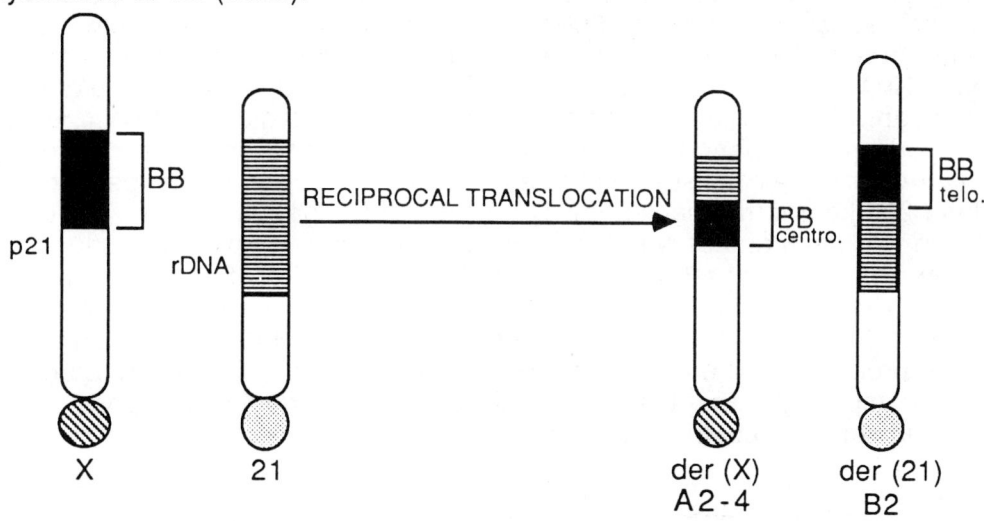

Figure 3

Sequences on the centromeric side of the deletion breakpoint hybridized to the 5.0 kb HindIII fragment in A2-4 and normal DNA but DNA from the telomeric side of the breakpoint hybridized to the 18 kb HindII band in normal and B2. A 4 kb HindIII+EcoRI fragment of the 10 kb BBJ-I insert hybridized only to the 5.0 kb HindIII band in A2-4 and normal DNA (Figure 2, step 4). It contained only sequences on the proximal side of the breakpoint but was not a unique sequence probe.

A unique sequence probe, BBJR.6, was isolated from the 4 kb HindIII+EcoRI fragment of BBJ-1 and was used to screen a 49,XXXXY, human genomic DNA library in λ DASH which we constructed. A set of overlapping phage clones were isolated and restriction mapped. These clones covered about 25 kb of genomic DNA including the proximal deletion breakpoint and the DXS140 (pERT55) locus (Figure 1). A unique probe, XH1.4, isolated from the most distal fragment of the 25 kb cloned, mapped approximately 15 kb telomeric from the deletion breakpoint. XH1.4 is deleted in BB and hybridizes to the X chromosome specifically.

IV. PULSED-FIELD GEL ELECTROPHORESIS (PFGE) MAPPING

The probes XH1.4 and a cDNA from the CGD locus (a gift from S. Orkin) were used to construct a detailed physical map of the proximal Xp21 region potentially containing the RP3 locus. These probes were hybridized to DNA from a lymphoblastoid cell line, derived from a single normal female, to avoid polymorphisms due to variations in methylation patterns between different cell lines. Infrequently cutting enzymes were used for mapping and each probe was successively hybridized to filters containing DNA digested with these enzymes singly and in combination.

Digestions performed using NotI alone showed hybridization of CGD and XH1.4 to distinct fragments of 600 kb and of >1000 kb respectively. The enzyme SfiI revealed a 205 kb fragment. This was the smallest band detected by both XH1.4 and CGD (Figure 4). When SfiI and NotI were used in combination, products of 40, 440 and 640 kb were detected by XH1.4 while CGD hybridized to bands of 165 and 640 kb. These single and double digestion results are consistent with both probes, XH1.4 and CGD, being on a common 205 kb SfiI fragment since 1) a common SfiI partial digestion product of 605 kb was seen and 2) NotI digestion separated the complete digestion SfiI band into fragments of 40 kb (XH1.4) and 165 kb (CGD), the sum of which yields 205 kb. The third SfiI site is predicted to lie approximately 400 kb proximal to the XH1.4 locus to generate the observed 440 kb partial/double digestion product (Figure 4). All the exons of the CGD cDNA used as a probe must lie completely within the SfiI 205 kb band as no additional bands were detected in single or double digestions.

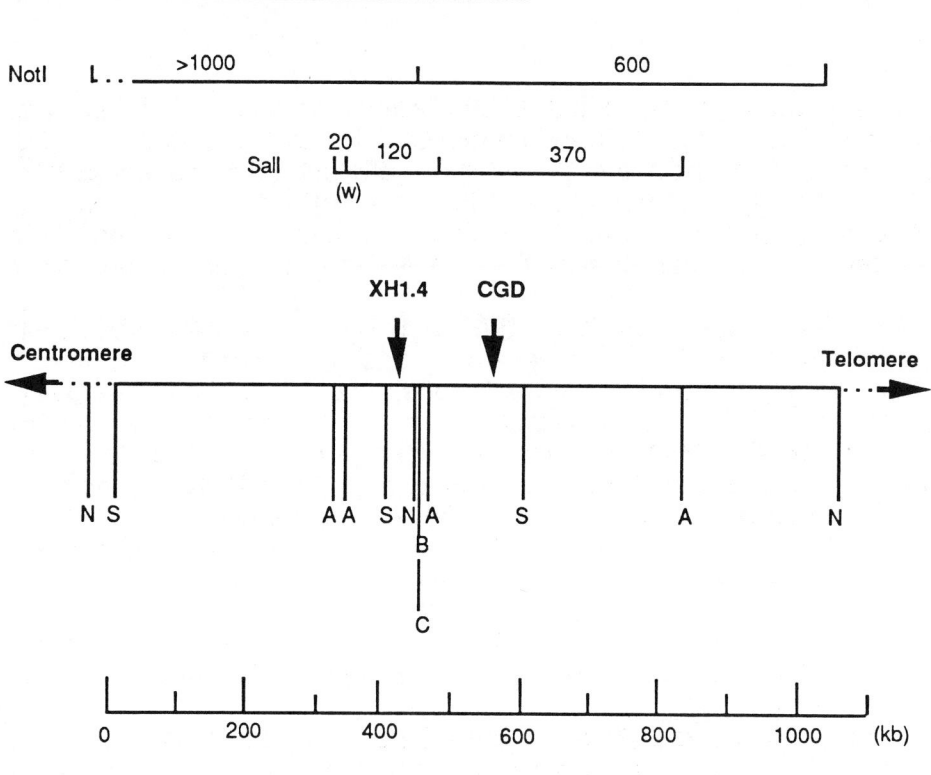

Figure 4

SalI digests proved particularly useful in detailed mapping of the region around the potential RP3 locus. Both probes recognized a "doublet", splitting into strong 490 kb and weak 510 kb bands. The other SalI products seen were a 370 kb band hybridizing to CGD and a pair of bands of 120 kb (intense) and 140 kb (weak) detected by XH1.4 (Fig. 4). These results suggested the probes were on adjacent SalI fragments and linked on common 490 kb and 510 partial digestion products. The SalI fragments of 120 kb and 140 kb detected by XH1.4 were reduced in size by approximately 10 kb when digested with NotI. In SalI+SfiI digests common partial digestion products of 255 kb (intense) and 275 kb (weak) were detected by both probes. Complete double digestion revealed 60 kb (XH1.4) and 145 kb (CGD) products, the sum of which suggests that a single SalI site is found within the common 205 kb SfiI fragment. The band intensity differences in the "doublet" seen initially with SalI digestion and repeatedly in double digestion with NotI and SfiI suggests a weakly cutting SalI site (w) 20 kb internal to another SalI site and argues against a SalI polymorphism (Figure 4).

The enzymes BssHII and SacII were also used singly and in combination with the other 3 enzymes. Briefly, the results are consistent with the placement of a BssHII site and a SacII site within the common 205 kb SfiI fragment and adjacent to one another and to the NotI site.

The interpretation of this data is summarized in the composite map in Figure 4 where S=SfiI, N=NotI, A=SalI B=BssHII and C=SacII. Individual enzyme maps could be co-aligned by the double digestion data. We have placed a BssHII and SacII site immediately adjacent to one another. This was consistent with SalI+BssHII and SalI+SacII digests that revealed a 105 kb band with XH1.4. Similarly SfiI+BssHII and SfiI+SacII digests revealed a band of 45 kb with XH1.4. The BssHII and SacII sites are therefore 45 kb from the SfiI site defining the common 205 kb fragment. A NotI site is approximately 5 kb proximal to these (XH1.4 mapped to a 40 kb SfiI+NotI digestion product). We suggest that these 3 sites (NotI, BssHII and SacII) indicate the presence of a CpG island in this region. The sites NotI, SacII and BssHII all contain CpG sequences, sequences frequently associated with the 5' end of genes.[24] The SalI site between XH1.4 and CGD is located approximately 15 kb telomeric to the BssHII and SacII sites (SfiI+SalI digestion revealed a band of 60 kb with XH1.4). Since this site effectively separates the CpG island (as different complete digestion products are detected with the probes used), it seems unlikely that the discovered CpG island is part of the CGD locus.

V. CLONING STRATEGIES

The maximum distance separating the CGD locus and XH1.4 can be no more than 200 kb since both these markers hybridize to a common SfiI fragment of 205 kb. All the exons of the CGD cDNA lie completely within this fragment and we have estimated the locus covers approximately 40 kb of genomic DNA based on the sum of the sizes of the restriction fragments detected by the cDNA probe on standard Southern blots. Therefore only 160 kb of DNA remains in which to search for the RP3 locus. In order to identify a gene which when defective results in XLRP we have continued chromosome walking from XH1.4 towards the 5' end of the CGD gene. The following criteria are being used to determine whether a cloned DNA fragment may contain candidate gene sequences: (i) detection of sequences which show evolutionary conservation, (ii) the presence of a CpG island (iii) expression in tissues affected by the disease as determined by Northern blot analysis or by isolation from cDNA libraries and (iv) sequencing of genomic fragments to detect possible open reading frames. The simplest first-step method for rapid screening of a large number of uncharacterized DNA fragments is the detection of sequence conservation by cross-species DNA hybridization at high stringency. The other criteria can then be applied to characterize selected sequences of interest. The effectiveness of this approach has been demonstrated in the successful cloning of the genes involved in DMD[4] and cystic fibrosis[7] and of a zinc-finger gene associated with Wilms tumours.[25]

As well as searching for sequences which may contain exons of a candidate gene we are looking for new RFLP's detected by the cloned segments of DNA isolated by chromosome walking. These are being used in further linkage analysis on our recombinant families to more precisely position the RP3 locus within the region analyzed in our long-range restriction map.

VI. REFERENCES

1. Ruddle, F.H., A new era in mammalian gene mapping: somatic cell genetics and recombinant DNA methodologies, *Nature* 294:115, 1981.
2. Orkin, S.H., Reverse genetics and human disease, Review, *Cell.* 47, 845, 1986.
3. Royer-Pokora, B., Kunkel, L.M., Monaco, A.M., Goff, S.G., Newgurger, P.E., Baehner, R.L., Cole,F.S., Curnette, J.T. and Orkin, S.H., Cloning the gene for an inherited human disorder - chronic granulomatous disease - on the basis of its chromosomal location. *Nature* 322: 32, 1986.
4. Monaco, A.P., Neve, R.L., Coletti-Feener, C., Bertelson, C.J., Kurnit, D.M., Kunkel, L.M. Isolation of candidate cDNAs for portions of the Duchenne muscular dystrophy gene. *Nature* 323: 646, 1986.
5. Burghes, A.H.M., Logan, C., Hu, X., Belfall, B., Worton, R.G. and Ray, P.N. A cDNA clone from the Duchenne/Becker muscular dystrophy gene. *Nature* 318:434, 1987.
6. Friend, S.H., Bernards, R., Rogel, S., Weinberg, R.A., Rapaport, J.M., Albert, D.M. and Dryja, T.P. A human DNA segment with properties of the gene that predisposes to retinoblastoma and osteosarcoma. *Nature* 323: 643, 1986.
7. Rommens, J.M., Zengerling-Lentes, S., Kerem, B., Melmer, G., Buchwald, M., Tsui, L-C. (). Physical localization of two DNA markers closely linked to the cystic fibrosis locus by pulsed-field gel electrophoresis. *Am. J. Hum. Genet.* 45: 932, 1989.
8. Bhattacharya, S.S., Wright, A.L., Clayton, J.F., Price, W.H., Phillips S, C.L., McKeown, C.M., Bird, J.M., Pearson, R.L., Southern, E.M., Evans, H.J. Close genetic linkage between X-linked retinitis pigmentosa and a recombinant DNA probe L1.28. *Nature* 309: 253, 1984.

9. Denton, M.J., Chen, J-D., Serravalle, S., Colley, P., Halliday, F.B. and Donald, J. Analysis of linkage relationships of X-linked retinitis pigmentosa with the following Xp loci: L1.28, OTC, 754, XJ1.1, pERT87, and C7. *Hum. Genet.* 78: 60, 1988.

10. Nussbaum, R.L., Lewis, R.A., Lesko, J.G. and Ferrell, R. Mapping of ophthalmological disease II. Linkage relationships of X-linked retinitis pigmentosa to X chromosome short arm markers. *Hum. Genet.* 70: 45, 1985.

11. Wirth, B., Denton, M.J., Chen, J-D., Neugebauer, M., Halliday, F.B., van Sschooneveld, M., Donald, J., Bleeker-Wagemakers, E.M., Pearson, P.L. and Gal, A. Short Communication: Two different genes for X-linked retinitis pigmentosa. *Genomics* 2: 263, 1988.

12. Musarella, M.A., Burghes, A., Anson-Cartwright, L., Mahtani, M.M., Argonza, R., Tsui L-C. and WORTON, R. Localization of the gene for X-linked recessive type of retinitis pigmentosa (XLRP) to Xp21 by linkage analysis. *Am. J. Hum. Genet.* 43: 484, 1988.

13. Musarella, M.A., Anson-Cartwright, L., Burghes, A., Worton, R.G., Lesko, J.G. and Nussbaum, R.L. Short Communication: Linkage analysis of a large Latin-American family with X-linked retinitis pigmentosa and metallic sheen in the heterozygote carrier. *Genomics* 4: 601, 1989.

14. Ott, J., Bhattacharya, S., Chen, J.D., Denton, M.J., Donald J., Dubay, C., Farrar, G.J., Fishman, G.A., Frey, D., Gal, A., Humphries, P., Jay B., Jay, M., Litt M., Machler, M., Musarella, M.A., Neugebauer, M., Nussbaum, R.L., Terwilliger, J.D., Weleber, R.G., Wirth, B., Wong, F., Worton, R.G. and Wright, A.F. Localizing multiple X-chromosome linked retinitis pigmentosa loci using multilocus homogeneity tests. *Proc. Natl. Acad. Sci. USA* 87: 701, 1990.

15. Lathrop, G.M. and Lalouel, J.M. Efficient computations in multipoint linkage analysis. *Am. J. Hum. Gen.* 42: 498, 1988.

16. Musarella, M.A., Anson-Cartwright, L., Leal, S.M., Gilbert, L.D., Worton, R.G., Fishman, G.A. and Ott, J. Multipoint linkage analysis and heterogeneity testing in twenty X-linked retinitis pigmentosa families. *Genomics* (in press).

17. Francke, U., Ochs, H.D., de Martinville, B., Giacalone, J., Lindgren, V., Disteche, C., Pagon, R.A., van Ommen, G-J.B., Pearson, R.L. and Wedgewood, R.J. Minor Xp21 chromosome deletion in a male associated with expression of Duchenne muscular dystrophy, chronic granulomatous disease, retinitis pigmentosa and McLeod syndrome. *Am. J. Hum. Genet.* 37: 250, 1985.

18. de Sainte-Basile, G., Bonler, M.C., Fischer, A., Carton, J., Dufler, J.L., Griselli, C. and Orkin, S.H. Xp21 DNA microdeletion in a patient with

chronic granulomatous disease, retinitis pigmentosa, and McLeod phenotype. *Hum. Genet.* 80: 85, 1988.

19.   van Oommen, G-J.B., Verkerk, J.M.H., Hofker, M.H., Monaco, A.D., Kunkel, L.M., Ray, P., Worton, R., Wieringa, B., Bakker, E. and Pearson, P.L. A physical map of 4 million bp around the Duchenne muscular dystrophy gene on the human X-chromosome. *Cell* 47: 499, 1986.

20.   Bertelson, C.J., Pogo A.O., Chadhuri, A., Marsh W.L., Redman, C.M., Banerjee, D., Symmans, W.A., Simon, T., Frey, D. and Kunkel, L.M. Localization of the McLeod locus (XK) within Xp21 by deletion analysis. *Am. J. Hum. Genet.* 42: 703, 1988.

21.   Burmeister, M., Monaco, A.P., Gillard, E.F., van Ommen, G-J.B., Affara, N.A., Ferguson-Smith, M.A., Kunkel, L.M. and Lehrach, H.   A 10-megabase physical map of human Xp21, including the Duchenne muscular dystrophy gene. *Genomics* 2: 189, 1988.

22.   Monaco, A.P., Bertelson, C.J., Coletti-Feener, C. and Kunkel, L.M. Localization and cloning of Xp21 deletion breakpoints involved in muscular dystrophy. *Hum. Genet.* 75: 221, 1987.

23.   Bodrug S.E., Burghes, A.H.M., Ray, P.M., Worton, R.G. Mapping of four translocation breakpoints within the Duchenne muscular dystrophy gene. *Genomics* 4: 101, 1989.

24.   Bird, A. P. CpG islands as gene markers in the vertebrate nucleus. *T.I.G.* 3 (12): 342, 1987.

25.   Gessler, M., Poustka, A., Cavenee, W., Neve, R.L., Orkin, S.H. and Bruns, G.A.P. Homozygous deletion in Wilms tumours of a zinc-finger gene identified by chromosome jumping. *Nature* 343:774, 1990.

USHER SYNDROME IN LOUISIANA

Mary Z. Pelias,[1] Richard J.H. Smith,[2]
Stephen P. Daiger,[3] and J. Fielding Hejtmancik[2]

[1] Louisiana State University Medical Center, New Orleans; [2] Baylor College of Medicine, Houston, Texas; [3] The University of Texas Health Science Center, Houston

I. INTRODUCTION

Usher syndrome (US) is a rare, autosomal recessive disorder characterized by congenital sensorineural hearing loss or deafness followed by the onset of retinitis pigmentosa in childhood or adolescence.[1] An unusually high incidence of this disease is found in the Acadian population of southwestern Louisiana. After several members of this group inquired about the possibility of determining carrier status for US, the search for a closely linked polymorphic genetic marker was undertaken. When possible linkage of the gene to a conventional protein marker on chromosome 4 was subsequently excluded by DNA marker studies,[2,3] the investigation was expanded to provide a systematic search of all chromosomes for a unique DNA marker that would indicate the presence of the deleterious allele. Recent identification of two families (from a total of 30) in which the affected offspring have clinical characteristics of a phenotypic variant of classic US has resulted in a removal of the data derived from these families into separate files for linkage analysis.[4]

II. POPULATION AT RISK

Southwestern Lousiana is the home of a large population of descendants of French Acadians who immigrated to the area in the latter third of the eighteenth century. Prior to their expulsion from Canada by the British in 1755, the Acadians had been established in Nova Scotia since the early years of the seventeenth century. After several years of wandering, some of the original Acadians began to arrive in Louisiana. Moving up the Mississippi River through New Orleans, they settled along the river banks and resumed their traditional agrarian lifestyle. Some families, however, who sought larger stretches of higher land, succeeded in traversing a formidable swamp basin that bisects the southern half of Louisiana. These settlers established communities along the bayous and in the prairies that lie considerably west of New Orleans.[5] The new settlements flourished, but they remained geographically isolated until well into the present century when highways across the state were paved and the petrochemical industry began to develop the rich oil and gas reserves along the Gulf of Mexico.

In addition to being physically isolated from other populations in Louisiana, the Acadians, or Cajuns, have also enjoyed a cultural isolation that to some extent persists into the present. Everyday life is focused on the church and the family. The Acadians are quietly devout in their Catholic faith. They have traditionally had large families and have cherished their many children. Their language has evolved from the French that their ancestors imported from rural France over three centuries ago, and this unique dialect has been the first language, both at home and in schools, until well past the middle of this century. As farmers and fishermen they have been attached for generations to the land and the waters of southern Louisiana, with the result that many families still reside within short distances of the homes of their ancestors. As musicians and story-tellers they revel in a singular joie-de-vivre that celebrates their contentment with themselves and their surroundings. And as hosts and guests the Cajuns prepare and appreciate a repertoire of regional cuisine that is unmatched. The Cajuns are a peaceful, unassuming people, slow to move and slow to change.[6]

In recent years science and technology have introduced new twists into Cajun life. Young people are now limiting the size of their families. New knowledge of the hereditary aspect of many health problems has been introduced in medical clinics, in school, and over the air waves. The general effect among many young adults has been an express interest in avoiding the birth of children with hereditary disabilities. The impetus for the search for carrier detection in Usher syndrome was generated among the families with affected children. With a reasonable assurance that the gene, or genes, or closely linked markers, will be identified, these families hope eventually to control the frequency with which affected children are born.[2]

III. LINKAGE STUDIES

Genealogical information about the US population in Louisiana was first amassed during the 1960's in a broad study of congenital deafness.[7] This information has been updated to include the last two generations of affected persons and their families. Most families are part of an immense kindred whose ancestry is traced to two couples who immigrated from France to Canada in 1636; the histories of an additional 18 nuclear families indicate probable relationship to older generations within the single large kindred.

With adequate pedigree information available, 30 nuclear families were initially selected for linkage studies. Samples of blood and saliva from 277 persons have been analyzed for 28 conventional polymorphic genetic marker systems. Linkage analyses of these data using sib-pair methods[6] as well as calculation of lod scores[7] indicated a possible linkage of the gene for US to the locus for group specific component (GC), which maps to the long arm of chromosome 4. The maximum lod score with GC, for equal male and female recombination fractions, was 1.41 at a recombination fraction of 0.17.[2]

The search for a DNA marker linked to the gene for US was initiated in collaboration with the National Retinitis Pigmentosa Foundation, Inc., and the Human Genetic Mutant Cell Repository in Camden, New Jersey, USA. DNA for these studies was prepared from transformed cell lines derived from blood samples submitted to the RP Cell Line Collection in the Cell Repository. These cell lines are available to the scientific community by contacting the Cell Repository.

Initial studies were undertaken with 15 probes specific to chromosome 4. Composite exclusion data indicated that the gene for US could be reliably excluded from approximately 80% of the length of that chromosome 4.[3] Subsequent multipoint linkage analyses with a total of 23 DNA probes have eliminated 50% of chromosome 6, 80% of chromosome 17, and 90% of chromosome 19 as possible sites for the location of the gene for US.[10]

Chromosome 2 is presently under investigation.

IV. CLINICAL HETEROGENEITY

Clinical heterogeneity in US has been recognized for many years,[11] and it has recently been investigated in five of the Acadian families.[4] In two families, 4 affected children out of a total of 10 offspring can be classified phenotypically as having US Type 2. These affected children have sufficient residual hearing that they benefit from the use of hearing aids and can communicate orally. They had normal developmental milestones, normal vestibular function, and normal motor skills. Affected children in three other families tested are clearly classified as having US Type 1. They are profoundly deaf and communicate only by signing. They also have delayed developmental milestones, abnormal vestibular function, and decreased motor skills. The Type 1 children tested are representative of the phenotypes of all affected children in the Acadian population except for the two families described above. The retinitis pigmentosa that appears in these families has a similar age of onset and slow clinical course across all affected families.

As a result of these new findings the marker data from the two Type 2 families have been separated from the data from the Type 1 families for purposes of genetic analysis. At this time, however, there is no new indication of a linkage for the US gene, or genes, in the Acadian population of Louisiana.

V. CONCLUSIONS

The Acadian population of Louisiana provides a unique opportunity to study Usher's syndrome and to develop scientific information that may be useful to the families who are coping with this form of deaf-blindness. On-going linkage studies have eliminated large portions of chromosomes 4, 6, 17, and 19 as possible sites of the Acadian gene, or genes. As our compendium of linkage information continues to grow, we can reasonably expect to identify markers, and eventually, the gene(s). While the demonstration of clinical heterogeneity in two Acadian families hints at the possibility of two genetic loci in this population, there is no clear evidence at this time to indicate the presence of more than one autosomal locus in this population.

REFERENCES

1. Vernon, M., Usher's syndrome - deafness and progressive blindness: clinical cases, prevention, theory, and literature survey, *J. Chron. Dis.*, 22, 133, 1969.

2. Pelias, M.Z., Lemoine, D.R., Kossar, A.L., Ward, L.J., Wilson, A.F., and Elston, R.C., Linkage studies in Usher's syndrome: analysis of an Acadian kindred in Louisiana, *Cytogenet. Cell Genet.*, 47, 111, 1988.

3. Smith, R.J.H., Holcomb, J.D., Daiger, S.P., Caskey, C.T, Pelias, M.Z., Alford, B.R., Fontenot, D.D., and Hejtmancik, J.F., Exclusion of Usher syyndrome from much of chromosome 4, *Cytogenet. Cell Genet.*, 50, 102, 1989.

4. Smith, R.J.H., Pelias, M.Z., Daiger, S.P., Herrera, C.A., Kimberling, W.J., and Hejtmancik, J.F., Clinical hererogeneity within the Acadian Usher population, in preparation, 1990.

5. Arsenault, B., *Histoire et Généalogie des Acadiens,* Éditions Leméac, Inc., Ottawa, 1978, vol. 1 and 6.

6. Rushton, W.F., *The Cajuns, from Acadia to Louisiana*, Farar Straus Giroux, New York, 1979, chap. 2, 3, 8-10.

7. Kloepfer, H.W., Laguaite, J.K., and McLaurin, J.W., The hereditary syndrome of congenital deafness and retinitis pigmentosa, *Laryngoscope*, 76, 850, 1966.

8. Elston, R.C., Sib pair screening tests for linkage, *Genet. Epidem.*, 1, 175, 1984.

9. Ott, J., *Analysis of Human Genetic Linkage*, Johns Hopkins University Press, Baltimore, 1985.

10. Smith, R.J.H., Herrera, C.A., Pelias, M.Z., Kimberling, W.J., Daiger, S.P., and Hejtmancik, J.F., Multipoint analysis of Usher syndrome: exclusion of chromosomes 6, 17, and 19, *Am. J. Hum. Genet.*, 45(4), A163, 1989.

11. McLeod, A.C., McConnell, F.E., Sweeny, A., Cooper, M.C. Nance, W.E., Clinical variation in Usher's syndrome, *Archs. Otolar.* 94, 321, 1971.

This research was generously supported by the National Retinitis Pigmentosa Foundation, Inc. and The George Gund Foundation, and by NIH Grant EY0714.

Address inquiries to:
Department of Biometry and Genetics
L.S.U. Medical Center
1901 Perdido Street
New Orleans, LA 70112 USA

"CATARACT COMPLICATED BY RETINITIS PIGMENTOSA"

Pannarale M.R., Rispoli E., Vingolo E.M., Pannarale L.,
Forte R. and Iannaccone A.

University of Rome "La Sapienza", Italy
Institute of Ophthalmology
Head: M.R. Pannarale

I. INTRODUCTION

We apply the definition of "complicated" to cataracts following other ocular affections, especially endo-ophtalmic phlogoses or chorioretinal degenerative disorders (chorioretinogenic cataracts).

Posterior Subcapsular Cataract (PSC) has been reported by various authors to be the most frequent form of opacity in patients affected with RP.[1-7]

The main purpose of this study is to emphasize the morphological and topographical aspects of cataracts in some patients examined in our Center and to evaluate the possible correlation between the occurrence of lens opacities in the groups considered here and the onset age of the first symptoms referrable to the disease.

II. MATERIALS AND METHODS

We studied 108 patients affected with RP who are continuously followed at the Center for Eredo-degenerative Retinal Disorders of the Institute of Ophthalmology of the University of Rome "La Sapienza". Of these, 57 (52.8%) were male and 51 (47.2%) female, going from 14 to 72 yrs. of age and with a mean age of 38.87 yrs. (± 13.026 SD).

Every patient had a thorough clinico-ophthalmological examination, including:
- accurate anamnesis to define the onset age;
- evaluation of the best corrected far and near visual acuity (V.A.) with the Snellen test card;
- central retinal Critical Fusion Frequency (CFF) for red and green with the best near correction;
- examination of the anterior segment (slit lamp biomicroscopy) and lens opacities and vitreal aspects study, evaluated with mydriatic iris;
- fundus examination by means of indirect binocular ophthalmoscopy and slit lamp biomicroscopy, to assess possible central retinal changes and to evaluate with particular emphasis the aspects of the optic disc, the occurrence of pigmentation, its density and its topographical aspects in the mid-peripheral area.

The patients also underwent instrumental diagnostic procedures, such as visual field testing by using the Goldmann's perimeter or computerized devices (e.g., Octopus 2000), electrofunctional analyses (with particular regard to massive ERG) and evaluation of lens opacities with retroillumination cameras (Neitz or Oxford) and Scheimpflug camera.[8]

Referring to the density and topography of the pigmentary pattern,[7] as assessed with indirect binocular ophthlmoscopic fundus examination, we have considered four groups of patients:

Group I: Typical Peripheral R.P. (70 patients, 40 of whom M and 30 F, mean age 36.8 yrs., range 14-72 yrs.);

Group II: Typical Peripheral R.P. with central involvment (24 patients, 11 M and 13 F, mean age 43.9 yrs., range 20-62 yrs.);

Group III: Atypical Sector R.P. (5 patients, 2 M and 3 F, mean age 34.2 yrs., range 20-47 yrs.);

Group IV: Atypical pauci-pigmentata R.P. (9 patients, 4 M and 5 F, mean age 43.8 yrs., range 30-53 yrs.).

Patients affected with syndromes associated to Retinitis Pigmentosa, such as Usher and Lawrence-Moon-Bardet-Biedl Syndromes, did not participate in this study.

We compared the occurence of Posterior Cortical Opacities (PCO) to the onset age of symptoms related to R.P., referring to three age ranges: 0-10 yrs., 11-20 yrs., > 20 yrs.

Data coming from this study were analized, from a statistical point of view, on the basis of the χ^2 test (tab. 2 x 2 with 1 degree of freedom) in order to verify the significance of the distributions.

III. RESULTS

In our sample Posterior Cortical Opacities (PCO) occurred in 70 patients out of 108 (64.8%).

The prevalence of this kind of opacity in the sub-groups considered in this study turned out to be the following:

Group I: 40 patients out of 70 (57.1%);
Group II: 23 patients out of 24 (95.8%);
Group III: 3 patients out of 5 (60%);
Group IV: 4 patients out of 9 (44.4%).

Table 1 illustrates the distribution of the above mentioned results obtained for Group I and II and their significance, evaluated on the basis of the χ^2 test (tab. 2 x 2 with 1 degree of freedom):

TABLE 1
Frequency distribution of PCOs

	Group I	Group II	
Presence	40	23	63
Absence	30	1	31
	70	24	94

Table 2 x 2
Degrees of freedom: 1
$\chi^2 = 12.10$
p<0.001

We considered the significance of the occurrence of lens opacities only in the first two groups since they include most of the patients who participated in this study (87%). The correlation between this parameter and the onset age revaeled to be as follows (Table 2):

TABLE 2

Correlation between occurrence of PCOs and onset age

	presence	absence
Group I		
0-10 yrs.	28%	25%
11-20 yrs.	10%	4%
>20 yrs.	19%	14%
Group II		
0-10 yrs.	62%	4%
11-20 yrs.	13%	-
>20 yrs.	21%	-

IV. DISCUSSION

Most of the Authors agree that chronic degenerative chorioretinal disorders (including R.P.) and co-existing PSCs have a different etiopathogenesis,[2,9] being the first ones the cause of the second ones (cataract intended as a secondary process).

In agreement with this point, in the context of our clinical research on R.P., we usually apply the definition of "complicated" to cataracts following other ocular affections, especially endo-ophtalmic phlogoses or chorioretinal degenerative disorders (the so-called "chorioretinogenic cataracts").

Present researches, in the attempt of clarifying the pathogenetic mechanism that may be the actual cause of this kind of opacities, are based on the above-mentioned hypotheses:

a) for an inflammatory pathogenesis, possible interferences on lens metabolism from substances produced during chronic chorioretinal degenerations are suggested (lysophosphatidylcholine),[10] as well as a possible release of reactive oxigen molecules - peroxides, hydroxide iones, etc. - by activated macrophages.[11,12] We believe this mechanism to be highly probable, on account of the peripheral macrophagic activation and the evidence for endovitreal activated macrophages pointed out in patients affected with Retinitis Pigmentosa;[13,14]

b) concerning the hypothesis of cataracts intended as a secondary phenomenon of chorio-retinal degenerations, an excessive peroxidation of membrane lipids with production of toxic aldehydes and lipidic radicals - such as docoexanoic acid - is considered as a possible etiopathogenetic factor.[11,15,16]

The most peculiar morphological aspects of cataracts complicated by chorio-retinal affections ("chorio-retinogenic" or "retinogenic" cataracts) entail opacities, described by other authors as "porous",[17] or "breadcrumb",[18] that we prefer to indicate as "spongioid". With this term we intend opacities localized in various lamellar layers in the region of the posterior pole, which tend to extend and deepen towards the nucleus, mainly following a sutural course (radiate opacities).

Eshagian et al.,[1,19] investigating the ultrastructure of lens subcapsular posterior areas in R.P., have demonstrated severe alterations of lenticular fibers - with areas of increased intracytoplasmatic density - and evidence of aberrant epithelial cells, resembling the anterior ones, which probably cause the formation of a neo-capsula, as it can be observed in the migration site of these cells.

Several authors have evaluated the prevalence of cataract in patients affected with RP. Heckenlively et al. reported on a sample of 291 patients also including, together with typical R.P. forms, atypical types, Usher's Syndrome, choroideremia and cone-rod degeneration cases; in this study the authors pointed out an overall occurrence of PSC in 41% of cases, with a lower prevalence for cone-rod degeneration and a higher prevalence for R.P. patients, particularly the autosomal dominant inheritance pattern.[2] Fishman et al. analyzing a sample of 338 patients, demonstrated a PSC in 53% of the subjects, showing a higher prevalence for the recessive X-linked pattern from autosomal recessive and sporadic ones.[4]

The prevalence of Posterior Cortical Opacities (PCO) pointed out for our sample (64.8%) is substantially different from values reported by other authors. In fact, it has to be considered that our case report included especially typical R.P. forms (87% of the total) together with atypical sectorial and pauci-pigmentatae R.P. ones, while associated syndromes and other inherited retinal degenerations were not taken into account. Conversely, Heckenlively et al. considered various clinical entities, pointing out only a 41% of opacities on 291 patients,[2] while Fishman et al. found a 53% on a group of patients made up only of typical R.P. cases.[4]

We also found a statistically significant correlation between the occurrence of PCOs and the ophthalmoscopic aspect of the ocular fundus. In fact, PCOs had a much higher prevalence in Group II (95.8%) than in Group I (57.1%) and, with regard to Group II, they were undoubtedly more frequent in subjects referring the onset of the first symptoms of the disease between 0 and 10 yrs. of age (62%).

These data demonstrate that cataract has to be considered as a major worsening factor for the visual performances of patients whose Visual Acuity is already profoundly compromised by a severe clinical status.

V. REFERENCES

1. Eshaghian J, Rafferty NS and Goossens W.: Ultrastructure of human cataract in retinitis pigmentosa. *Arch. Ophthalmol.* 98: 2227, 1980.

2. Heckenlively JR: The frequency of posterior subcapsular cataract in the hereditary retinal degenerations. *Am. J. Ophthalmol.* 93: 733, 1982.

3. Marmor MF, Aguirre G, Arden G, Berson E, Birch DG et al. : Retinitis Pigmentosa, a symposium on terminology and methods of examination. *Ophthalmology* 90: 126, 1983.

4. Fishman GA, Anderson RJ and Lourenco P.: Prevalence of posterior subcapsular lens opacities in patients with retinitis pigmentosa. *Br. J. Ophthalmol.* 69: 263, 1985.

5. Heckenlively JR: *Retinitis Pigmentosa.* JB Lippincott, Philadelphia, 1988.

6. Pagon PA: Retinitis Pigmentosa (Major Review). *Surv. Ophthalmol.* 33 (3):137, 1988.

7. Jimenez-Sierra JM,Ogden TE and Van Boemel GB: *Inherited retinal diseases. A diagnostic guide.* The C. V. Mosby Company, St. Louis, 1989.

8. Pannarale MR, Vingolo EM, Pannarale L, Feher JM, Arrico L, Perdicchi A. and Ricci A: La cataratta complicata da miopia. Presented at the 5th IACRR International Congress, Rome, November 17-19, 1989.

9. Merin S.: Cataract formation in retinitis pigmentosa.*Birth Defects Orig Art Ser* 18 (6): 187, 1981.

10. Cotlier E, Basking M, Kresca L: Effects of lysophosphatidyl choline and phospholipase A on the lens. *Invest Ophthalmol Vis Sci* 14: 697, 1975.

11. Zigler JS, Bodaness RS, Gery I and Kinoshita JH: Effects of lipid peroxidation products on the rat lens in organ culture: a possible mechanism of cataract initiation in retinal degenerative disease. *Arch Biochem and Bioph* 225: 149, 1983.

12. Miglior M: Le cataratte correlabili a malattie oculari (cataratte complicate). Presented at 2nd IACRR International Congress, Cefalù (Palermo, Italy) October 17-19, 1986.

13. Vingolo EM, De Marco G, Modugno FP, Perdicchi A, Ippoliti F and Pannarale MR: Reattività immunitaria cellulomediata nella Retinite Pigmentosa. *Boll Ocul* 67(6): 1037, 1988.

14. Newsome DA, Michels RG: Detection of lymphocytes in the vitreous gel of patients with retinitis pigmentosa. *Am. J. Ophthalmol.* 105: 596, 1988.

15. Goosey JS, Tuan WM and Garcia CA: A lipid peroxidative mechanism for posterior subcapsular cataract formation in the rabbit: a possible model for cataract formation in tapetoretinal diseases. *Invest Ophthalmol Vis Sci* 25: 608, 1984.

16. Simonelli F, Nesti A, Pensa M, Romano L, Savastano S, Rinaldi E and Auricchio G: Lipid peroxidation and human cataractogenesis in diabetes and severe myopia. *Exp Eye Res* 49: 181, 1989.

17. Nordmann J: *Biologie du cristallin.* Masson Et., 355, 1954.

18. Duke-Elder S: *System of ophthalmology.* XI, 210, 1969.

19. Eshaghian J: Human posterior subcapsular cataracts. *Trans. Ophthalmol. Soc. UK* 102: 364, 1982.

R.P. ITALIA ASSOCIATION REFERENCE CENTRE OF MILAN: FIRST RESULTS

A. Porta, G. Staurenghi, C. Pierrottet, F. Piattoni*, V. Gualandri*, L. Troiano°, M. Del Bo°

Department of Ophthalmology, University of Milan, Italy
* Institute of Human Genetics, University of Milan, Italy
° Institute of Audiology, University of Milan, Italy

INTRODUCTION

F.I.A.R.P. (Federation of Italian Retinitis Pigmentosa Associations) was founded in 1990 to coordinate all regional Associations, to establish a common protocol, to start a National Registry, to fund in research laboratories under the guidance of a scientific advisory board.
This report covers the 18 months of activity, prior to F.I.A.R.P. foundation, of the R.P. Italia Association which collected patients with Retinitis Pigmentosa (RP) from Lombardy.
The organization is devised so that, whatever the first referral centre, the patient is rapidly referred to the other reference centres (Table 1).

Table 1. Management of a new RP patient

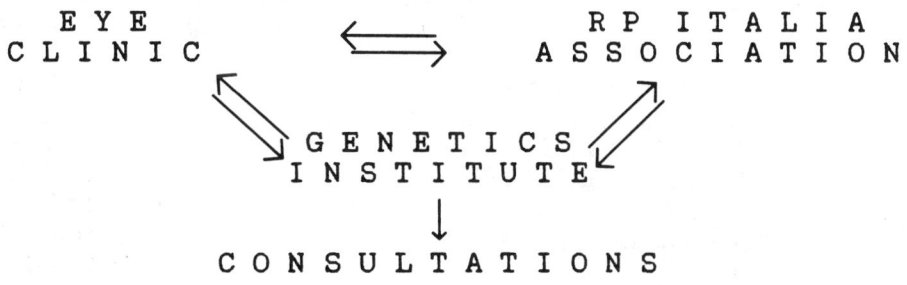

PATIENTS AND METHODS

During the last 18 months, 171 patients with Retinitis Pigmentosa were referred to the Department of Ophthalmology of the University of Milan and examined according to a protocol based on the one proposed by Heckenlively in 1988 (1) (medical and ocular history; best corrected visual acuity; colour vision testing; Goldmann kinetic perimetry; dark adaptation test; biomicroscopy of the anterior segment; applanation tonometry; dark and light adapted ERG; fundus colour photography; fluorescein angiography).
During the same period, 172 unrelated probands were referred to the Institute of Human Genetics of the University of Milan for genetic counseling: family and personal medical hystories were obtained, a complete pedigree (up to third degree relatives) drawn, a priori risks evaluated and at-risk individuals identified for further examination.
Affected subjects were referred to the Audiology Institute of the University of Milan for audiometric testing (air and bone conduction threshold determination, 250-8000 Hz; speech reception threshold determination; middle ear acoustic immitance measurements; vestibular function investigations). When necessary medical, neurologic, and pediatric consultations were asked.

RESULTS

Table 2 shows the results in the 171 ophthalmologic patients. Patients were classified according to the diagnostic criteria as reported in the literature.

Table 2. Ophthalmologic patients

171 pts	96 m.	mean age 37.37 yrs.
	75 f.	ranging 0.33 - 83

* 141 PRIMARY FORMS
  - 3 LEBER AMAUROSIS
  - 8 JUVENILE RP
  - 2 EARLY ONSET RP
  - 64 ROD-CONE RP
  - 57 CONE-ROD RP
  - 1 PPRPRE RP
  - 4 CHOROIDEREMIA
  - 2 UNKNOWN RP TYPE

* 30 SECONDARY FORMS
  - 7 USHER I
  - 8 USHER II
  - 9 L.M.B.B.
  - 2 ALSTROM
  - 1 SAL-MAIN
  - 3 UNKNOWN

Patients with classical primary RP were divided into the Cone-rod (CR) and Rod-cone (RC) subtypes on the basis of direct and indirect criteria, as reported in Table 3.

Table 3. Cone-rod and Rod-cone type inclusion criteria
CONE-ROD
Direct: Cone   ERG   more   severely   affected   than   Rod
           ERG, with both Cone and Rod ERGs abnormal
Indirect: Final Rod threshold of 2.00 log units
           or less of elevation
           Visual field ring scotomata between 5°-30° and
           concentric rings in later stages
           Usually, history of late onset night blindness
           (>20 yrs)
ROD-CONE
Direct: Rod   ERG more severely affected than Cone ERG,
           with both Cone and Rod ERGs abnormal
Indirect: Final Rods threshold of 3.5 log units or greater
           Visual field large jumps in sensitivity among
           isopters as well as ring scotomata between 30°-
           50°
           Usually, history of early onset night blindness
           (<20 yrs)

Indirect criteria apply to RP patients with an advanced
disease (unrecordable ERG, visual field less than 10° and
Dark Adaptation Test showing severe night blindness).
For 115 out of 121 patients with CR or RC RP, complete
ophthalmologic history and data were obtained: results are
shown in Table 4.

**Table 4. Analysis of 115 patients with complete
ophthalmologic history and data**

	total		CR		RC	
pts	115	(43)	57	(25)	58	(18)
males	61	(21)	29	(12)	32	(9)
females	54	(22)	28	(13)	26	(9)
mean age	40.56	(39.55)	41.89	(39.99)	39.24	(38.95)
1st symt.	16.46	(20.12)	21.69	(24.72)	11.32	(13.72)
night bl.	16.07	(17.23)	20.43	(19.68)	11.79	(13.83)
duration	24.16	(18.80)	19.67	(14.29)	28.57	(25.00)

*) in brackets data regarding patients with recordable ERG.

The 172 unrelated patients who were referred for genetic
counseling were classified according to clinical diagnosis
and inheritance pattern (Table 5). Primary forms of RP with
no recognizable AD or X-L R inheritance were further
divided into 16 different classes on the basis of pedigree
analysis.

Table 5. Genetic distribution of 172 families who were referred for genetic counseling

Autosomal recessive RP (AR)	115
AR1 (sporadic male)	18
AR2 (sporadic female)	15
AR3 (male, same parental birthplace)	16
AR4 (female, same parental birthplace)	22
AR5 (2 males or more)	3
AR6 (2 females or more)	0
AR7 (2 males, same parental birthplace)	1
AR8 (2 females, same parental birthplace)	0
AR9 (male, consanguineous parents)	6
AR10 (female, consanguineous parents)	10
AR11 (male and female)	3
AR12 (2 males, consanguineous parents)	2
AR13 (2 females, consanguineous parents)	1
AR14 (male and female, same parental birthplace)	7
AR15 (male and female, consanguineous parents)	2
BAR16 (more than 2 affected of different sexes)	9
Autosomal recessive RP syndromes (ARS)	29
Autosomal dominant RP (AD)	9
X-linked recessive RP (X-LR	5
Inheritance pattern to be defined (IPD)	6
Other retinal degenerations	8
TOTAL	172

males   96   females   76

Complete ophthalmologic and genetic data were obtained for 83 families with primary and secondary RP (Table 6).

Table 6. Complete ophthalmologic and genetic data in 83 families with primary and secondary RP

Autosomal recessive RP				n	RC	CR
				62	28	34
	n	RC	CR	n	RC	CR
AR1	14	7	7	AR2	8	4	4
AR3	9	5	4	AR4	6	2	4
AR5	0	0	0	AR6	0	0	0
AR7	0	0	0	AR8	0	0	0
AR9	5	3	2	AR10	9	2	7
AR11	2	0	2	AR12	1	1	0
AR13	0	0	0	AR14	6	3	3
AR15	0	0	0	AR16	2	1	1

	n	RC	CR
Autosomal recessive RP syndromes	13	9	4
Autosomal dominant RP	3	2	1
X-linked recessive RP	1	0	1
Inheritance pattern to be defined	4	3	1
TOTAL	83	42	41

Segregation analysis was performed on the 63 families with primary RP and no evidence of AD or X-L R transmission (Table 7) by means of the Single complete ascertainment and the Multiple incomplete ascertainment methods ("Sibs" and "Singles" methods) (2,3).

Table 7. Primary non AD/X-LR forms sibships

	probands		brothers		sisters	
	M	F	U	A	U	A
AR1	14	0	5	0	5	0
AR2	0	8	7	0	7	0
AR3	9	0	3	0	7	0
AR4	0	6	4	0	4	0
AR5	0	0	0	0	0	0
AR6	0	0	0	0	0	0
AR7	0	0	0	0	0	0
AR8	0	0	0	0	0	0
AR9	5	0	3	0	3	0
AR10	0	10	8	0	9	0
AR11	1	1	2	1	4	3
AR12	1	0	1	1	1	1
AR13	0	0	0	0	0	0
AR14	4	1	10	2	10	4
AR15	0	0	0	0	0	0
AR16	0	2	0	2	0	3
TOTAL	34	28	43	6	49	8
	62		49		57	

Singles: 52/62   (83.9%)

Audiologic examination was carried out on 47 patients with primary RP.

DISCUSSION AND CONCLUSIONS

Patients (mean age 40.56 yrs) were evaluated long after the onset of symptoms (mean duration of disease: 24 yrs) so that about 65% of our present cases have advanced forms with unrecordable ERG: in these patients RC or CR patterns are to be desumed from indirect criteria. Onset is earlier and duration is longer in patients with a RC form than in patients with a CR form.
Audiologic examination on 47 patients with primary RP

identified 18 patients (38%) with a sensorineural hearing loss ranging from mild (20-40 dB) to severe (70-90 dB). No significant correlation of the hearing loss with the disease duration was found: the 18 patients with hearing impairment seem to cluster in advanced age (50-65 yrs).
A genetic classification of patients was performed on the basis of pedigree analysis.
A high proportion of simplex cases (i.e. with only one affected individual) was found (83.9%). Clear autosomal dominant (direct vertical transmission in at least 2 generations) or X-linked recessive (multiple affected males in the maternal tree) transmission was found in a minority of cases (3/83 and 1/83). Autosomal recessive transmission seems fairly probable in 25/83 families (classes AR7 to AR16). Due to the small size of the studied population no definite conclusion about proportions of known genetic types of RP can yet be reached.
Population ascertainment approaches single selection: with the "single" and "sib" methods the maximum likelyhood estimate of segregation ratio ranges between 0.13 and 0.21. The federation of national RP Associations in F.I.A.R.P. will permit to enlarge the clinical population and to perform a more thorough genetic analysis of RP distribution.

References

1. J.R. Heckenlively: Retinitis Pigmentosa. Philadelphia, J.B. Lippincott, 1988
2. C.C. Li, N. Mantel: A simple method of estimating the segregation ratio under complete ascertainment. Amer. J. Hum. Genet., 20, 61-68, 1968
3. R.A. Fisher: The effect of methods of ascertainment upon the estimation of frequencies. Ann. Eugen. (Lond), 6, 13-25, 1934

Acknowledgments

We are indebted to Italian Retinitis Pigmentosa of Milan fur the supply and management of the patients examined in the present study.

Linkage Analysis of Northern Ireland Autosomal Dominant Retinitis Pigmentosa Families

R.Redmond[*], B.Page[*] & A.E.Hughes[+]

Departments of Ophthalmology[*] & Medical Genetics[+], Queen's University, Belfast.

Summary

Four Autosomal Dominant Retinitis Pigmentosa (ADRP) families in Northern Ireland have been investigated using the DNA markers D3S47 (C17) and D3S14 (R208). Preliminary DNA linkage data are reported on. Two families, one with early-onset symptoms and the other with late-onset symptoms show possible tight linkage with D3S14. The practicality of disease classification based on age-of-onset and electrophysiological findings is discussed.

Introduction & Background

Retinitis Pigmentosa is a significant cause of visual morbidity in the Northern Ireland population younger than 65 (Bryars[1], Page[2]). 15% of affected individuals in the province can be clearly identified as comforming to the autosomal dominant mode of inheritance (ADRP).

Attempts have been made to accurately sub-classify ADRP, based on the following criteria:

History : age of onset of nyctalopia

Examination : visual acuity[3], visual field loss and retinal pigment distribution

Fundus reflectometry : measurement of the distribution and concentration of photoreceptor rhodopsin[4]

Electrophysiology : scotopic (dark-adapted, rod photoreceptors) and photopic (light adapted, cone photoreceptors) ERG

e.g.   (Massof & Finkelstein[5])

Type 1 -   early & diffuse loss of rod function; later regionalised cone function loss.

Type 2 -   regionalised & combined loss of rod & cone function or :   (Fishman et al.[6])

> *Type 1 -*   severe, diffuse pigment changes with concentric depression of
> visual fields and flat ERG.

> *Type 2 -*   regional pigment changes and corresponding field changes,
> abnormal but preserved cone receptor ERG response.

(other Fishman 'Types' exist with,in practice, considerable clinical overlap between the types.

With the 'split' that such classifications imply, it is natural to attempt to correlate such apparent phenotypic heterogeneity with genetic heterogeneity. This correlation can now be attempted using the tools of DNA linkage analysis, which in the case of ADRP has been stimulated by the recent report of tight linkage between the DNA probe C17 (D3S47) and the chromosome 3q gene locus for a single Type 1 (Massof), early-onset, Irish family (McWilliam et al.[7], $LOD_{MAX} = 14.7$, theta = 0). A second probe, R208 (D3S14), was also linked. There are no Northern Ireland ADRP pedigrees as extensive as that studied by McWilliam et al.[7] Nevertheless, of the pedigrees most promising for linkage studies, the results and preliminary evaluations of 4 are presented.

Methods

DNA was extracted from the venous blood of affected individuals and other key relatives (Jeanpierre[8]). 5 microgram DNA aliquots were digested with MspI and BglII restriction enzymes with subsequent agarose gel electrophoresis and vacuum blotting onto Hybond N+ filters (Amersham). 50 ng aliquots of probes C17 and R208 were labelled with [^{32}P]-dCTP using the random hexanucleotide primer method of Feinberg and Vogelstein[9]. Unincorporated nucleotides were eliminated by passage through a Sephadex G50 column. Probes were pre-annealed with human placental DNA before hybridisation to filters (see Ingelhearn et al.[10]). Allele systems revealed by autoradiography are listed in Table 1.

Table 1

		Enzyme	
		MspI	**BglII**
Probe Name	**C17**	A1 - 14 kb A2 - 12.3	
	R208	B1 - 6.7 kb B2 - 5.3 B3 - 4.0, 2.9	A1 -7.0 kb A2 -3.6,3.2

LOD scores were calculated using the MLINK program of Linkage (v5,03).

Results and Comments

Scored allele patterns (haplotypes) are shown below each individual member in the partial pedigrees (Figures ADRP 1,2,3 and 4). Haplotype numbers in order are MspI/C17, MspI/R208 and BglII/R208.

ADRP 1 :   Analysis 'suggests' tight linkage ($LOD_{MAX}=0.215$ at theta = 0) with the 2,3,2 haplotype present in all 5 'proven-affected' members. The average age of nyctalopia is at 25 years for this family (Range 23-28). Female III_1 is currently asymptomatic at age 13, though she does manifest retinal pigment changes and has a subnormal ERG. I_2 died at the age of 56, and a history from immediate kin strongly suggests that he was asymptomatic. It is presumed that the disease is non-penetrant for this individual. Unaffected male II_3 is 45 years old and asymptomatic. As he bears the 2,3,2 haplotype, the question remains whether he is a 'form fruste', a recombinant or a true non-penetrant. Penetrance for this family is 5/6 = 83%

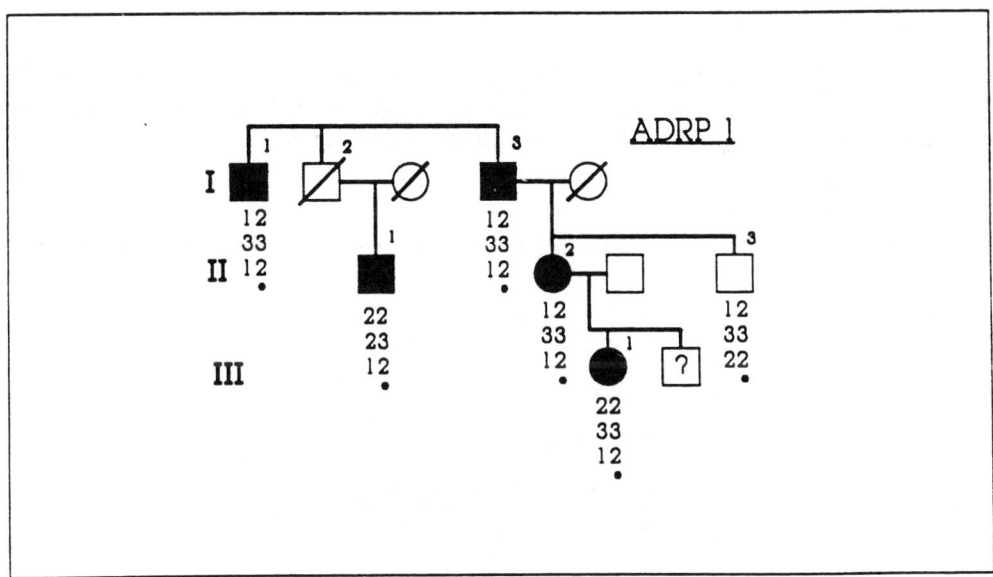

ADRP 2 :   No evidence for linkage. Unaffected male (III$_1$) has the 2,3,1 haplotype in common with his father and two affected siblings. Two other affected siblings (III$_{2,5}$) do not bear the 2,3,1 haplotype. The father of II$_5$ remains asymptomatic, but presumably bears the same disease gene as his deceased sister, therefore : Penetrance = 8/9 = 89%

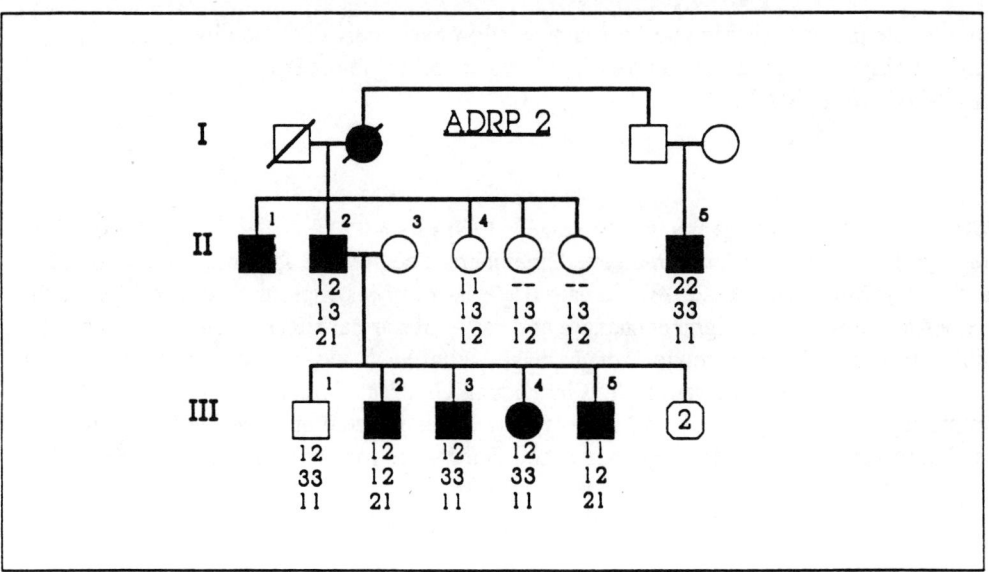

ADRP 3 :   DNA analysis reveals a 2,3,2 haplotype in the 3 affected siblings in generation II, again 'suggesting' tight linkage. Childhood onset was common to these three. Analysis of further members of this family is necessary to reach more significant conclusions about linkage.

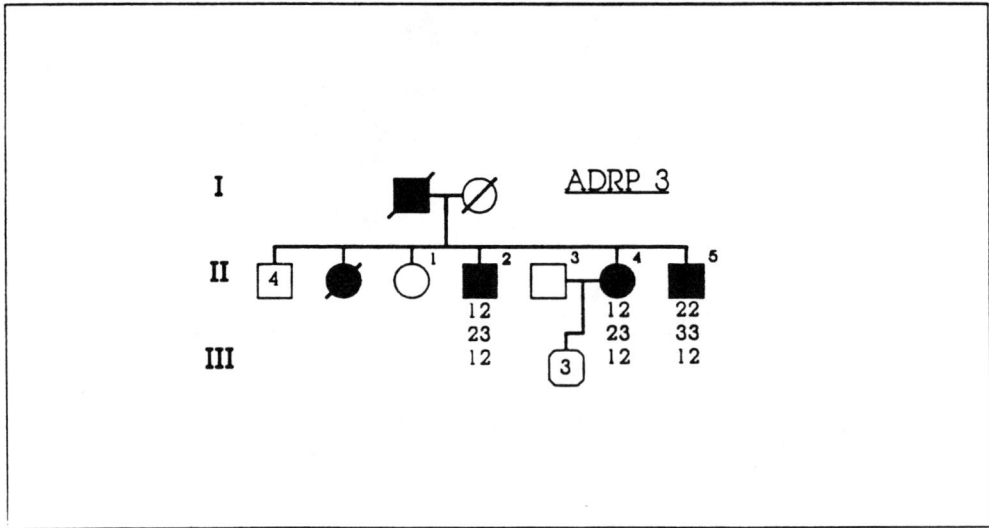

ADRP 4 : Linkage is excluded in this family. The eldest affected female and her affected offspring share a 1,1,2 haplotype, and the remaining sisters in the first generation and two daughters ($I_{3,5}$ and $II_{4,5}$) share a 1,2,1 haplotype. These haplotypes originate in different grandparents, hence conclusions of linkage based on I_1 being the only recombinant in this family are not valid.

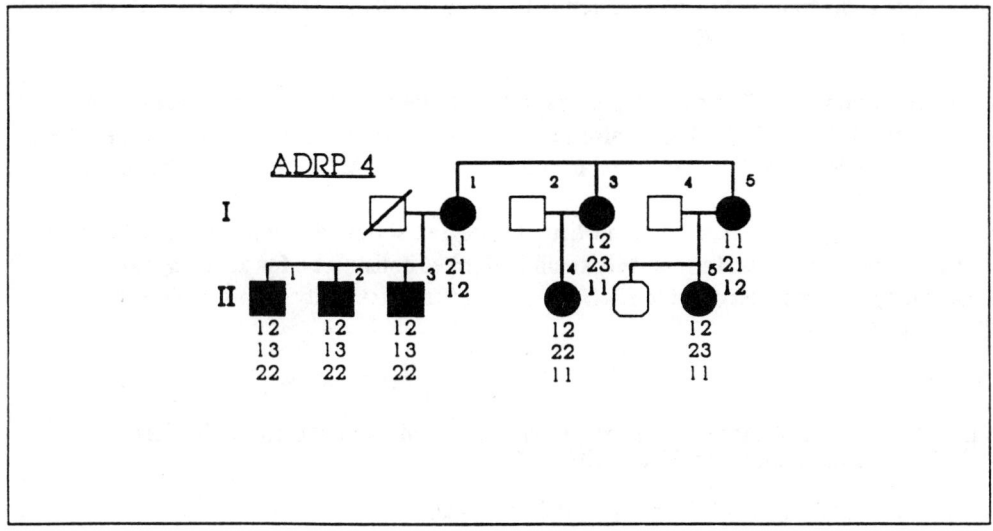

Table 2

	LOD$_{MAX}$ (D3S14)	Theta	Penetrance	Av. Age of Onset	Age Range
ADRP 1	0.22	0	83%	25	23 - 28
ADRP 2	0	.5	89%	16	7-25
ADRP 3	0.15	0	100%	7	7-8
ADRP 4	0.01	.4	100%	21	10-30

Discussion

Study of ADRP families in Northern Ireland raises several points of interest.

■ DNA linkage analysis on small pedigrees suggests tight linkage of D3S14 (R208) to the disease gene in both early and late-onset families (ADRP 1 & 3). In other families studied, the gene causing ADRP is not linked to this locus.

■ These typical ADRP pedigrees demonstrate the wide range for age of onset of nyctalopia that is frequently encountered, and the possibility of reduced penetrance. The early-onset Irish family (TCDM1 - as reported by McWilliam et al.[7]) was 100% penetrant. ADRP 1 is late-onset with penetrance reduced to 83%

■ Both ADRP 1 and 3 families show a 2,3,2 haplotype linked in coupling with the disease allele. The same D3S47 (C17) allele is also linked in the previously reported TCDM1 kindred, raising the suggestion of a 'founder' effect for all Irish cases of ADRP linked to this locus.

■ Designation of Type 1 or Type 2 to a particular pedigree should depend upon ERG changes as well as 'age of onset' data. In relatively small pedigrees considered for analysis, most individuals may have non-recordable ERGs, reducing the practicality of this form of sub-classification.

References

1 Bryars JH, Archer DB. Aetiologic survey of visually handicapped children in Northern Ireland. Trans. Ophthalmol. Soc. UK. 97:26-29, 1977.

2 Page B. MD Thesis. Queen's University, Belfast, 1988.

3 Farber MD, Fishman GA, Weiss RA. Autosomal dominantly inherited retinitis pigmentosa : Visual loss by subtype. Arch. Ophthalmol. 103:524-528, 1985.

4 Fitzke FW. Clinical Psychophysics. Eye 2(Supplement):S233-S241, 1988.

5 Massof RW, Finkelstein D. Two forms of autosomal dominant primary retinitis pigmentosa . Doc. Ophthalmol. 51:289-346, 1981.

6 Fishman GA, Alexander KR, Anderson RJ. Autosomal dominant retinitis pigmentosa. A method of classification. Arch. Ophthalmol. 103:366-374, 1985.

7 McWilliam P, Farrar GJ, Kenna P et al. Autosomal dominant retinitis pigmentosa (ADRP): Localisation of an ADRP gene to the long arm of chromosome 3. Genomics 5:619-622, 1989.

8 Jeanpierre M. A rapid method for the purification of DNA from blood. Nucl. Acids Res. 15:9611, 1987.

9 Feinberg AP, Vogelstein B. A technique for radiolabelling DNA restriction endonuclease fragments to high specific activity. Anal. Biochem. 132:6-13, 1983.

10 Inglehearn CF, Jay M, Lester DH et al. No evidence for linkage between late onset autosomal dominant retinitis pigmentosa and chromosome 3 locus D3S47 (C17): Evidence for genetic heterogeneity. Genomics 6:168-173, 1990.

TAPETO RETINAL DYSTROPHY AND MENTAL RETARDATION

Mette Warburg *, Ole Sjö *, Lisbeth Tranebjærg **

* Gentofte Hospital, Division of Paediatric Ophthalmology and Handicaps; ** The John F. Kennedy Institute, Dept. of Medical Genetics, Gl. Landevej 7, DK-2600 Glostrup, Denmark.

INTRODUCTION

People with mental retardation (MR) may have tapeto-retinal dystrophies (TRD) just like all other people, but there are no large surveys of the types of TRD observed among them. The aim of this study was to describe the various types of TRD observed within a very large group of MR patients seen in our clinic.

MATERIAL

Ascertainment was retrospective. The case notes of all patients with M.R. and TRD or cone dystrophy seen in the clinic for the last 15 years were examined. The patients derived from several series. The majority were patients with MR from our referral area comprising a population of approximately 1 mio people. Visually impaired patients with MR from other areas were also referred to this clinic, and those with TRD are part of the material. Some patients were examined elsewhere, and the case notes were evaluated by the first author. Finally, a census of all MR and visually handicapped children from 1976 (1) gave information about patients from our own referral area and other counties.

CLINICAL EXAMINATIONS

All patients had a paediatric or internal medical examination before referral. Audiological and dental examinations were obtained when needed. Visual acuity was measured with Østerberg or LH pictographic charts or Teller acuity charts. Almost all patients could be examined in a slitlamp. The retina was observed with direct and indirect opthalmoscopy with and without a contact lens. A retinoscopic refraction was performed when autorefraction was impossible.

Many of the patients did not talk. Hemeralopia was judged by making the patient walk about in strongly reduced illumination, if the patient was able to walk; but many patients were bound to wheelchairs. Colour vision was examined by AO-HRR tables, Ishihara tables, Farnsworth 15 hue dichotomous or Lanthony desaturated buttons. If impossible, the patient was

asked to match small sugar balls of different desaturated colours.
ERG was obtained as described elsewhere (2). The oldest ERG curves were obtained with the Karpe method. High resolution chromosome analyses were performed on MTX-synchronized, RBA-banded chromosomes (3).

RESULTS

There were 3000 case notes concerning mentally retarded patients. TRD was assessed in 114 persons (4%). The disorders observed are shown in Table 1.

TABLE 1
Mental Retardation and Tapeto-retinal Dystrophy

Laurence Moon Bardet Biedl	26
Batten (Spielmeyer-Vogt)	20
Miscellaneous, identified	25
Chromosomal aberrations (causal)	3
Multiplex	9
Unidentified simplex non-syndromic RP	9
TRD MR Hearing loss	6
Unidentified syndromic RP	16
Total	114

IDENTIFIED SYNDROMES
There were 26 patients with the Bardet-Biedl syndrome and 20 with Batten disease. A number of miscellaneous identified syndromes with TRD were observed as shown in Table 2.
Four patients with mucopolysaccharidoses and one patient with Niemann-Pick disease were enzymatically identified. The patients with cystathioninuria, Menkes disease, and infantile Refsum diseases were also assessed biochemically.
Three patients belonged to the group of ceroid lipofuscinoses. Two of them had the Bielchowsky-Jansky syndrome which was identified clinically in one case and by autopsy in the other. The patient with the Santavuori-Hagberg syndrome was seen together with Dr. Santavuori. Senior-Löken, Leber congenital amaurosis and myotonic dystrophy were also clinical diagnoses. The Fukuyama syndrome was identified by muscle biopsy. The patient with the Cohen syndrome has been described previously (4).
Fibroblasts were cultured from some of the patients and examined for plasmalogen biosynthesis; plasma was examined for cholesterol and abnormalities of lipoprotein in order to detect peroxisomal dysfunction, but all samples were normal.

CHROMOSOMAL ABERRATIONS
Six patients with various chromosomal aberrations were found. Trisomy 21 was observed in two patients with rod-cone dystrophy. A translocation 13;14 was present in a patient with Leber congenital amaurosis. His healthy father and sister had

TABLE 2
Miscellaneous Identified Syndromes with MR-RP

No of patients	Syndrome
4	Mucopolysaccharidoses: Hunter, Sanfilippo A, Hurler-Scheie, Maroteaux-Lamy
5	Usher
3	Leber congenital amaurosis
3	Lipofuscinoses: Bielschowsky-Jansky, Santavuori
3	Myotonic dystrophy
2	Fukuyama congenital muscular dystrophy
1	Niemann-Pick
1	Cystathioninuria
1	Menkes disease
1	Infantile Refsum
1	Cohen syndrome

the same translocation. A boy had a translocation 1;6 and a cone dystrophy, and a young man had a deletion 18q221 together with a cone-rod dystrophy (2,5,6). There was a young man with mosaic trisomy 9 and a rod-cone dystrophy.

MULTIPLEX CASES
    Three sibships consisted of affected males only. In each sibship at least one of the affected males had a normal high resolution karyotype.
    In the fourth sibship the proband had cryptorchidism, cleft palate, and umbilical hernia. The karyotype was normal. A sister and brother had RP without other impairments.
    One of the patients with trisomy 21 was an affected member of a family with autosomal dominant RP.

SIMPLEX (SPORADIC) CASES
    Simplex cases were observed in four males and five females with normal karyotypes. ERG was extinguished in 5 patients, a rod-cone dystrophy was found in 4 individuals, and a cone dystrophy was observed in one. They had no malformations, and a specific diagnosis was not established.

UNIDENTIFIED SYNDROMES
    There were 6 patients with an association of TRD, hearing impairment, and neurological disorders. In no cases were familial cases known.
    In 16 patients the syndromes could not be further delineated. The patients had serious neurologic complications, epilepsia being the most common (8 cases); spastic palsy was also often seen. Most of these patients were examined for abnormalities of serum and urinary aminoacids, mucopolysaccharides, and lysosomal enzymes. Phytanic acid was examined in special cases. No diagnostic results were obtained.

DISCUSSION

IDENTIFIED SYNDROMES

Among our patients 4% had TRD. The prevalence of TRD among MR people, however, cannot be deduced from this study due to the unknown number of MR patients from whom the patients were drawn, and due to the difficulties in assessment by non-ophthalmologists, which will reduce the patients referred to the clinic. Furthermore some of the patients believed to be retarded were probably not so.

Few patients with moderate or severe MR see an ophthalmologist, and it is even more rare that ERG examinations can be obtained. If the patients do not talk, or if they have no idea about how well everybody else sees, they have no opportunity of demanding an eye examination.

It is a risk that the staff believes that patients with unidentified low vision have very low competence. Such misunderstanding was supposedly involved when 5 patients with Usher's disease had been notified as MR. They all came from an institution which was situated furthest away from schools for deaf and blind people. Some of them were presumably understimulated and put into custodial care for want of better arrangements.

Batten (Spielmeyer-Vogt) disease is the most common lipofuscinosis, and at the time of the census in 1976 there were 20 cases known to us. These children are not mentally handicapped until about 7-9 years of age. Patients with the Batten and Bardet-Biedl diseases are cared for elsewhere in this country, and the patients were included only due to the census.

Patients with the Bardet-Biedl syndrome are usually not retarded or only mildly so (7). In spite of this 26 had been notified to the care of MR children. Bardet-Biedl syndrome is therefore the most important differential diagnostic problem in ophthalmology when TRD is found in a supposedly MR child.

ERG changes in Hurler, Scheie, Hunter and Sanfilippo syndromes have been described (8) and this study, while Maroteaux-Lamy syndrome is supposed not to show such alterations. In our patient, excretion of chondroitin sulfate established the diagnosis, but TRD was only clinically assessed, and ERG was not performed. It is thought that the retinal involvement in the mucopolysaccharidoses is due to excess storage of MPS in the interphotoreceptor matrix.

It is of importance to staff and family to understand that a number of metabolic disorders eventually lead to visual impairment as well as progressive debility. This information will explain how to approach and handle the patients, and how to prevent difficulties associated with tunnel vision and low contrast sensitivity.

LCA was diagnosed in four patients who had severe visual impairment since infancy, low or attenuated ERG, and no signs of specific disorders. There were three other patients who had infantile TRD; one of them was a member of a family in which TRD appeared in infancy in one child and later in others. Two children had moderate hearing impairment together with their congenital TRD. Their syndromes were not identified.

MR is common in children with LCA (9), and this has given rise to a delineation into complicated and uncomplicated LCA (8).

It is unknown if this clinical delineation corresponds to genetic and microbiological entities since the biochemical defect(s) in LCA is/are unknown.

When LCA is considered among MR patients, the most important differential diagnosis is cortical visual impairment. Since the latter is a common disorder among severely retarded children, access to ERG is important. LCA is an autosomal recessive disease, while cortical visual impairment is a sequel to massive acquired cerebral lesions. There will therefore be great differences in genetic counselling and prognosis in the two diseases.

Two patients with myotonic dystrophy had clinical signs of TRD, in the third patient ERG was extinguished. Subnormal ERG is often but not invariably found in patients with myotonic dystrophy (10).

In two boys Fukuyama congenital muscular dystrophy (CMD) was found histologically, and ERG showed rod dystrophy. These patients show similarities with the Finnish muscle-eye-brain syndrome (11,12). The syndrome has not been definitively delineated. It has been proposed that CMD with cerebral malformations is identical with the Walker-Warburg syndrome (13,14), but there is no absolute agreement (15).

CHROMOSOMAL DISORDERS

The prevalence of TRD associated with presumed causal chromosomal aberrations was small (2%) in this population as compared to the prevalence of chromosomal aberrations in unselected groups of MR persons (18.8%), and compared to the prevalence of chromosomal aberrations (10%) in MR patients with microphthalmos and coloboma (16,17).

Trisomy 21 was observed in two patients, and are presumably accidental findings. A translocation 13;14 was present in the healthy father and sister of the affected boy with LCA. This translocation is very common and was assumed to be unrelated to the retinal disorder. The translocation 1;6 and the deletion 18q221 suggest map positions of a cone dystrophy to the distal end of 6q and of a cone-rod dystrophy to 18q211 (2,5,6). The relation between mosaic trisomy 9 and TRD is obscure.

SIMPLEX AND MULTIPLEX CASES

TRD was familial in five families. In 3 families only males were affected, but the mothers showed no signs of being carriers. There were no other affected relatives. High resolution karyotypes showed no deletions in these males.

The third family was special. One of the affected males had hydrocephalus, one of patients had infantile TRD and the third had ordinary juvenile RP. High resolution kayotypes were normal and consanguinity was absent. Biochemical abnormalities were not disclosed, and a precise syndromological diagnosis is obscure.

In the fourth family the non-retarded sister and brother had ordinary juvenile RP. The MR brother had several malformations which might have an eitiology separate from the RP.

In the fifth family autosomal dominant RP was present. The patient with mosaic trisomy 21 was the only known person with Down syndrome in the family, and we regard the association as coincidental.

UNIDENTIFIED SYNDROMES
    Although the majority of TRD in the MR population can be identified, there are syndromes still waiting to be delineated. We saw 6 patients with hearing impairment, various malformations and TRD. We also observed 16 patients with TRD, epilepsia, spastic palsy or other signs of CNS pathology. It is possible that some of the unidentified syndromes are mitochondrial disorders, and we will explore this possibility.

CONCLUSIONS

    A survey of tapeto-retinal dystrophy (TRD) among individuals with mental retardation (MR) has not been described before. Among 3000 MR patients who had ophthalmological examinations, we have observed 114 patients with TRD. While 74 (65%) of the patients had a variety of rare identifiable syndromes, there were 31 (27%) in whom no precise differential diagnosis was obtained, and 9 whose classification was only by their mode of inheritance. Causal chromosomal aberrations were observed in 3 patients. These cases suggest the chromosomal loci of a cone dystrophy to the distal part of 6q and a cone-rod dystrophy to 18q221 (2,5,6). The unclassifiable disorders were syndromes with TRD, epilepsia, hearing loss and spastic palsy. The study is not informative for the prevalence of TRD among MR people.

ACKNOWLEDGEMENTS
This work was supported in part by grants from the Velux Foundation, the Danish Foundation to Combat Eye Diseases and Blindness, the Hvass Foundation, Fonden til Lægevidenskabens Fremme (The AP Møller Foundation), and the Eye Foundation from The Danish Association of the Blind.

REFERENCES

1.   Warburg M., Frederiksen P., Rattleff J., Blindness among 7700 mentally retarded children in Denmark. In Smith V. & Keen J. (eds) Visual Handicap in Children. Clinics in Developmental Medicine No 73. Spastics International Med. Publ. with W. Heinemann Med. Books, pp 68-75. London, 1979.

2.   Warburg M., Sjö O., Tranebjærg L., Deletion mapping of a retinal cone-rod dystrophy: assignment to 18q211, *Am. J. Med. Genet.*, in press.

3.   Beck B., Mikkelsen M., Chromosomes in the Cornelia de Lange syndrome, *Hum. Genet.* 59: 271-276, 1981

4.   Warburg M., Pedersen S.A., Hørlyk H., The Cohen syndrome, *Ophthalmic Paediatr. Genet.* 11: 7-13, 1990.

5.   Tranebjærg L., Sjø O., Warburg M., Retinal cone dystrophy and mental retardation associated with a de novo balanced translocation 1;6(q44;q27), *Ophthalmic Paediatr. Genet.* 7: 167-173, 1986.

6.   Tranebjærg L., Warburg M., Sjö O., Abnormal karyotypes and retinal dystrophies. Communication to the first international conference on human genetics and anthropology. Cairo 1989.

7.   Green J.S., Parfrey P.S., Harnett J.D., Farid N.R., Cramer
      B.C., Johnson G., Heath O. et al, The cardinal mainifesta-
      tions of Bardet-Biedl syndrome, a form of Laurence-Moon-
      Biedl syndrome, New Engl. J. Med. 321; 15: 1002-1009, 1989.
8.   Heckenlively J.R., Retinitis Pigmentosa. J.B. Lippincott,
      Philadelphia, 1988.
9.   Schroeder R,, Mets M.B., Maumenee I.H., Leber's congenital
      amaurosis, Arch. Ophthalmol. 105: 356-359, 1987.
10.   Kert E., Ganes T., Clinical and electrophysiological ab-
      normalities in the visual system in myotonic dystrophy,
      Ophthalmologica 198: 95-102, 1989.
11.   Raitta C., Lamminen M., Santavuori P., Leisti J., Ophthalm-
      ological findings in a new syndrome with muscle, eye and
      brain involvement, Acta Ophthalmol. (Copenh.) 56: 465-
      472,1978.
12.   Santavuori P., Somer H., Sainio K., Rapola J., Kruus S.,
      Nikitin T., Ketonen L., Leisti J., Muscle-Eye-Brain disease
      (MEB), Brain Dev. 11: 147-153, 1989.
13.   Dobyns W.B., Pagon R.A., Armstrong D., Curry C.J.R., Green-
      berg F., Grix A., Holmes L.B. et al, Diagnostic criteria
      for Walker-Warburg syndrome, Amer. J. Med. Genet. 32: 195-
      210, 1989.
14.   Leyten Q.H., Fons J.M., Gabreëls J.M., Renier W.O., Ter
      Laak H.J., Sengers   R.C.A., Mullaart R.A., Congenital
      muscular dystrophy, J. Pediatr. 115; 214-221, 1989.
15.   Santavuori P., Pihko H., Sainio K., Lappi M., Somer H.,
      Haltia M., Raitta C., Ketonen L., Leisti J., Muscle-eye-
      brain disease and Walker-Warburg syndrome, Amer. J. Med.
      Genet.. 36: 371-372, 1990.
16.   Warburg M., Diagnostic precision in microphthalmos and
      coloboma of heterogeneous origin, Birth Def. Orig. Art.
      Series 18: 31-50, 1982.
17.   Rasmussen K., Nielsen J., Dahl G., The prevalence of chrom-
      osome abnormalities among mentally retarded persons in a
      geographically delimited area of Denmark, Clin. Genet. 22:
      244-255, 1982.

PERSPECTIVES ON HUMAN GENOME MAPPING

Robert Williamson, Department of Molecular Genetics, St. Mary's Hospital Medical School, University of London, London W2 IPG.

SUMMARY

A complete map of the human genome already exists, although in some parts the probes are widely spaced. During the next five to ten years, the map will be completed by the collaborative efforts of many groups internationally, making use of the new techniques of molecular genetics and computer science. There will be three major applications of the human gene map. There will be many new gene products which are discovered from the map, and which can be mutated so as to alter or target their function. Gene probes delineated by their map position will be used for prenatal and presymptomatic diagnosis and carrier testing (when requested) of all serious single gene diseases. Finally, and perhaps most exciting, the diversity of mutations causing severe conditions such as RP, as well as the common pathologies of midlife such as heart disease, mental illness and cancer in mid or later life, will be elucidated. While the development of this genetic map does not pose any new or unique medical or ethical problems, its very scale will highlight certain personal and societal dilemmas which have previously only been confronted in special and restricted situations. In spite of this, the establishment of the human gene map should be seen as a fundamentally and totally positive step which will allow progress to new major advances in preventive medicine.

INTRODUCTION

It seems remarkable that the first human gene analysis related to an inherited disease (alpha-thalassaemia) using DNA techniques was only reported in 1974 by my colleague Sergio Ottolenghi (Glasgow) and Y. W. Kan (San Francisco); the human globin genes were cloned in 1978 by Bernie Forget (Yale) and Peter Little (St. Mary's London). For the first few years after these pioneering steps, molecular genetics was applied exclusively to the study of human diseases where there is simple Mendelian inheritance, and where the defective protein was known, as for thalassaemia and sickle cell disease, phenylketonuria and Lesch-

Nyhan syndrome. However, soon after Kan reported the first polymorphisms which could be detected by a cloned human gene, Solomon and Bodmer pointed out that these DNA variants represented a resource for gene mapping with the potential to supercede existing marker systems.

RESTRICTION FRAGMENT LENGTH POLYMORPHISMS (RFLPs)

The polymorphism identified by Kan is not in, but adjacent to, the beta-globin gene-specific probe which was used to visualise it, and is due to the presence or absence of a specific DNA sequence at one site in the gene. This sequence is one that is recognised by a restriction enzyme, and when it is mutated a DNA fragment of a different length is generated. Of course, the difference can only be visualised if a gene specific probe is available which can pair precisely with the sequence at the locus where the mutation occurs. This type of polymorphism is known as an RFLP; several million of these exist between any two people (it was estimated by Jeffreys that there is one base change occurring at random every few hundred base pairs throughout the human genome, though this is probably an overestimate) and for the ten years after their first description in 1978 by Kan, they were the most frequently used of the DNA polymorphisms.

Studies were first performed in families in which inherited diseases occurred, especially the approximately 700 single gene mutations where the protein that is altered is known. The great majority of these mutated genes have now been cloned, using the mapping functions of gene-specific probes, and the mutations have been determined by sequence for at least some affected individuals.

Two general points arise from the results of this work. First, there are many diseases - even the simplest genetic conditions - which vary in the way they present. A person can be severely or mildly affected, or one organ can be more or less affected as against another. This sometimes reflects mutations in different genes, but it seems that it is much more common to find that the same gene is mutated in every clinical case, with the actual site of the base change or deletion within the gene differing, leading to different effects on the corresponding protein. Second, there is no rule as to how many different mutations in a gene occur to cause the same disease in different families. In the case of genes on the X-chromosome, most mutations are different, as would be expected. However, even for autosomes some diseases (such as cystic fibrosis) have a single mutation which causes the majority of cases, while others, also recessive (such as phenylketonuria) have a multiplicity of changes. There appear to be few generalisations which hold for Mendelian diseases as a whole.

GENE DIAGNOSIS

What has been the impact of the isolation of cloned genes

corresponding to the mutated sequences for most of the Mendelian diseases, and the identification of many of the specific changes which cause pathology? As soon as the gene is identified, DNA analysis of any individual within a family, or (when the mutation is found in most of the individuals affected) a population, can immediately give the "genotype" - whether a person is carrying the mutated gene or not, and in how many copies. This allows DNA diagnosis either of the disease or for carriers. Since the DNA in any tissue of the body (apart from the egg or sperm cells) is the same, this diagnosis is independent of which tissue is studied, and of whether or not the person has yet shown symptoms.

Therefore, DNA testing is essentially presymptomatic, in that it is fully independent of any clinical information. For most diseases, it is completely accurate. It is particularly suitable for prenatal diagnosis (in several modes), and also for predicting whether someone will develop a single gene disease later in life (as for late onset dominant disorders like Huntington's chorea or myotonic dystrophy).

Prenatal diagnosis is already available for most single gene diseases which are serious and where the protein that is mutated is known (leading to the isolation of the gene sequence and the definition of the mutation). I will assume that those at this symposium share my view that the decision as to whether to have, or not to have, a handicapped child is one which is fundamentally up to the parents, and that medical and scientific services have a responsibility to provide information allowing that decision to be taken as early as possible, and with as much knowledge as possible. Whatever the decision, it deserves support from society. Once termination of pregnancy is legal within a society for a case of severe handicap, there are no new ethical issues (only personal advantages to the mother-to-be and her partner) if the information is provided with greater accuracy or earlier in the pregnancy.

The availability of gene maps, probes and diagnostics has, however, transformed aspects of the information that is available. First, carrier testing using DNA is cheap (probably of the order of $2 per test), non - invasive (using a scrape from the inside of the mouth, rather than a blood sample), and totally accurate. It may be possible to carry out DNA tests on the very small number of fetal cells that are found in the maternal circulation, rather than having to take a fetal sample by chorion or amniocentesis. It is certainly possible to do DNA analysis on a four or eight cell embryo after fertilisation in vitro (by IVF), and may even be possible to analyse egg cells prior to fertilisation, to determine which carry and which do not carry a mutation! These applications are only just over the horizon, and will be attempted during the next year or two in clinical practice. While I do not feel that they alter the ethical situation (since I believe in choice), certainly the availability of pre-fertilisation analysis of oocytes might alter the attitude of those who have the view that "life starts at the moment of fertilisation. Only fertilisation which is known to lead to an unaffected fetus could take place if this technique is offered.

REVERSE GENETICS - FROM LINKAGE TO MUTATION

For most clinical conditions, things are not as simple as for the diseases mentioned above - even if they are Mendelian. Often, the inheritance proves that a single gene is involved, but the protein that is affected is unknown, as for example, in Huntington's chorea. Ten years ago, it seemed unlikely that it would be possible to understand diseases such as these using molecular genetics. However, a decade ago, acting on the advice in the Solomon/Bodmer letter, several groups began to implement the strategy now known as reverse genetics.

Because recombination for any human chromosome occurs rarely during meiosis, a small number of probes are sufficient to define the whole sequence of DNA, from top to bottom. As few as 200 or so highly informative, polymorphic DNA markers are sufficient for the whole human chromosome set, giving a complete map of the human genome. Each marker can then be followed through families in which a disease occurs, and coinheritance between a disease and one allele (variant) of a DNA probe studied. Coinheritance will only occur if the cloned DNA is close to the mutation causing the disease. This linkage analysis was first performed by Kay Davies at St. Mary's London for Duchenne muscular dystrophy, and later used by three groups (Toronto, St. Mary's London and Salt Lake City) to locate cystic fibrosis to human chromosome 7.

DNA variants (RFLPs) used to be found by pure chance (and a lot of hard and expensive research); fortunately, Weber and Litt have recently shown that variants are particularly plentiful near to some features of the DNA landscape, especially runs of repeats of the dinucleotide (AC) and next to the repetitive sequence family known as Alu. The details of these sequences are unimportant; the significance is that any region of the genome can now be "marked" for inheritance studies quickly and efficiently, and all families that are studied are "informative" for gene probes.

The results of reverse genetics studies on single gene defects are well known. The defining of the dystrophin gene on the human X chromosome by Lou Kunkel (Boston) was a true landmark - this gene is mutated so as to cause Duchenne muscular dystrophy, and the most significant aspect is that dystrophin is a <u>new</u> gene which had been completely unknown before the use of reverse genetics. Instead of using classical biochemical techniques to identify and characterise the origin of diseases, the new molecular genetics techniques are comprehensive and reductionist, in that they require no knowledge other than a clinical diagnosis and a family which is affected through which DNA sequences can be followed. The most recent well publicised application of this technology was by Lap-Chee Tsui (Toronto), who defined the gene mutations causing cystic fibrosis, once again in a gene which was unknown prior to the application of reverse genetics.

THE IMPLICATIONS FOR SINGLE GENE DISEASES

There are about 4,000 diseases which are caused by a single gene defect, but where the protein mutation is unknown. These will gradually be understood as our gene map becomes more comprehensive. Although many of these conditions are rare, as a clinical group they account for a great deal of pathology. Probably fully half of paediatric bed days in hospital in first world countries result from genetic diseases, with the major implications for the affected children, their families and the health care systems of our society. The isolation of the mutated genes, and the attendant understanding of causation, will mean that those at risk of having children affected by severe inherited disease will have the option of prenatal diagnosis early in pregnancy, and those who decide to continue with such pregnancies will have access to better treatment.

COMMON POLYGENETIC AND MULTIFACTORIAL DISEASES

Important as single gene diseases are, the major health burdens in European societies are due to conditions that affect men and women in middle and later life - heart disease, cancer, diabetes, arthritis, Alzheimer's disease, mental illness. None of these are "genetic" in the sense that cystic fibrosis or muscular dystrophy is, yet all have a genetic as well as an environmental component. Some families exist in which a disease occurs very frequently, but more often, there is a general familial tendency to get a disease, but non-Mendelian inheritance. (Every lay person knows that there are families in which heart disease, or cancer, or mental illness, seems to "run in the family", although not inherited in a strict sense.) In my view, the single most important outcome of molecular genetics during the next decade will be the new insights that it offers us in understanding these multifactorial diseases of later life.

Of these diseases, there are some which are truly genetic, in that risk is primarily determined by inheritance, but where the time and severity of onset can be modified by behaviour. Perhaps the best example is coronary artery disease, of the type caused by high blood cholesterol. A few people have a catastrophic genetic defect (usually in the gene coding for the cell surface receptor recognising the protein that carries cholesterol around the blood) which causes early onset heart disease. A few have a catastrophic life style (butter, drink, cigarettes) which causes early onset heart disease. But most of those who develop heart disease do so because of a mixture of the two - they inherit genes which predispose to high circulating cholesterol, and then also increase this risk by their behaviour. The great advantage of gene analysis will be to pinpoint those at high risk, so they can have the option of modifying their behaviour in the more or less certain knowledge that it really will make a difference.

THE RARE PARADIGMAL FAMILY

There are many other ways to use gene mapping to understand the environment. My colleagues Gudrun Moore and Al Ivens (St. Mary's London) have studied a large cleft palate family from Iceland in which a single gene in the middle of the long arm of the X-chromosome determines who gets the defect. They have located the mutation to a two million base pair stretch of DNA. But cleft palate is not usually genetic at all; it seems to be caused either by environmental agents or pure chance. Why bother with this rare family?

We feel that large families in which conditions which are not usually genetic segregate as Mendelian traits are exceptionally valuable, since they can allow us to understand the mechanism that causes the pathology. In the case of cleft palate, we hope that by understanding the gene mutation, we will also gain insight into the mechanisms of action of the environmental agents that can cause cleft palate, and create a safer environment in this way.

THE ECONOMICS OF DNA ANALYSIS

There is no doubt that gene analysis began as a costly technology, for the most part in the United States and the most advanced countries in Europe. Moreover, all of the early techniques required expensive equipment (such as ultracentrifuges and radioactive counters), even more expensive consumables (radioactive isotopes and restriction enzymes), and skilled staff who could use these. Technological advances, fortunately, do not <u>always</u> lead to increased costs; in the case of human gene analysis, the combination of polymerase gene amplification (PCR) and other new techniques which do away with the need for ultracentrifugation and radioactive isotopes have transformed not only the cost, but also the accessibility, of the technology.

Our laboratory has now run courses on the use of PCR for gene analysis for cystic fibrosis for the European Community and the World Health Organisation; among those attending have been scientists from most of the countries of Eastern Europe, several countries in Latin America, and a few in Africa and Asia. These have <u>all,</u> without exception, been able to start gene analysis on their population in order to help prevent this severe disease. While these countries are, for the most part, second (rather than third) world, in that they have reliable services and trained staff, it has been impressive how universal this experience has been. Moreover, for the most part, the technology works without spending much "hard currency"; the only import is the enzyme which is used to amplify the DNA.

GENE ISOLATION AND NEW TREATMENTS

However, the impact of gene isolation goes beyond diagnosis and also will lead to improved treatment. At present, there are many diseases where rational treatment cannot be started because the underlying nature of the disease is not known at the molecular level. This is most clear in the second large group of inherited diseases, those which have a known Mendelian inheritance (i.e., only a single gene is mutated) but the defect and the gene are not known. The models for this have been cystic fibrosis (autosomal recessive), Huntington's chorea (autosomal dominant), and Duchenne muscular dystrophy (X - linked). It is only through increased knowledge of the genes involved that any advance in treatment will be possible.

What sorts of advances in treatment might legitimately be expected? First and foremost, traditional pharmacological approaches. Now that we know that cystic fibrosis is caused by a mutation in the nucleotide binding site of the CF transmembrane regulator, drugs can be designed which will attempt to restore normal function. Although there is a great deal of discussion about the exciting future possibilities of specific somatic gene therapies, the fact that time-tried approaches also depend upon these molecular genetics data should not be lost sight of.

In conclusion, for Retinitis pigmentosa, as for many other inherited diseases where more than one mutation can cause a variable phenotype, the availability of the human gene map, together with techniques for identifying mutations and examining them in model systems, should lead to better diagnosis, prevention and treatment during the next ten to twenty years.

ACKNOWLEDGEMENTS: Many colleagues have helped in our work over the years; I would particularly thank Charles Coutelle, Kay Davies and Steve Humphries for helping me to form views on the wider aspects of these issues; the views are, of course, my own. Our scientific work has been generously supported by the Medical Research Council and the Cystic Fibrosis Research Trust for many years. I have not given references in this paper; I am sure that anyone who wishes to follow up the specific work mentioned will be able to find appropriate papers from the literature quoted in any standard text or review. This article is based in part upon a previous talk given in Stockholm in March 1990, at a conference on "Trends in Biotechnology".

INDEX